Contents

Preface

Nursing Management by Dee Ann Gillies has gained prominence as a nursing management text in graduate schools, RN to BSN programs, and generic BSN programs as well as proving to be a valuable resource to nurse managers. The broad-based theoretical yet applied content has been updated in the third edition to reflect the many changes in the health care delivery system and in nursing management. This *Manual* provides supportive materials and up-to-date applications to nursing management faculty as they share the ever changing and challenging aspects of nursing management.

The diversity of backgrounds of the users of Gillies' *Nursing Management* text has been considered in the writing of the *Manual.* The test questions provided for each chapter are classified either as requiring beginning levels of knowledge and/or comprehension or as requiring a higher level of learning of application, analysis, or synthesis. The classification of the test questions allows faculty to select an evaluation level which best matches the student group. The test questions, with answers noted, are also referenced to text content.

Educational research has long demonstrated the lasting value of active, experiential and discovery learning over passive, "spoon fed" learning. Experiential and discovery learning activity ideas presented in the following pages aid the student in becoming an active rather than a passive learner, make learning more interesting, allow greater growing of the individual student, and require greater flexibility from the faculty. Helpful discussion ideas, group activities, and case situations presented in the *Manual* draw upon hypothetical health care facilities which represent the gamut of health care services to provide realistic situations requiring active student participation and critical thinking. The use of fictitious health care facilities, situations and people in community and longterm care as well as acute care hospitals will aid faculty in preparing nursing managers for the diversity of health care settings. The accompanying Content Summary provides a quick reference to the activity content of each of the chapters of this *Manual.*

To further assist faculty, the *Manual* includes chapter outlines to provide content focus at a glance; a list of key terms, several overhead suggestions to use in the classroom; student handouts and worksheets. Chapter outlines and key terms are helpful student study tools. Faculty may reproduce chapter outlines and key terms for distribution to students. The activities include assignment ideas which may be used with individual chapters, or may serve as topics from which students may choose for a term paper. The material provided in this *Manual* will help make the teaching of nursing management a relevant, exciting, and rewarding experience.

Suzanne Galliford, RN, Ed.D.

Content Summary

Chapter	Intro	Key Terms	Outline	Discussion	Group Activities	Assignments	OHS & Figs	Questions & Answers	Pg.
1	x	x	x	xx	xx	xx	x	26	1
2	x	x	x	x	x	xx		18	11
3	x	x	x	x	xx		x	13	19
4	x	x	x		x	x		25	27
5	x	x	x	x	xx			44	35
6	x	x	x	x			x	17	45
7	x	x	x	x		x	xx	38	53
8	x	x	x	x	x	xx	x	22	65
9	x	x	x		xx	x		27	73
10	x	x	x		x	x		25	83
11	x	x	x		x	xx	x	18	91
12	x	x	x		x	x	x	30	101
13	x	x	x		x	x	x	26	111
14	x	x	x	x	x			19	121
15	x	x	x	x	xxx	x		21	127
16	x		x	x	xx			14	137
17	x	x	x		xx		x	28	145
18	x	x	x	xx	xx	x	x	44	155
19	x	x	x	xx		x		41	167
20	x	x	x	xx		x		30	179
21	x	x	x	xx	x		x	26	189
22	x	x	x	x	xxxxx			30	199
23	x	x	x	xx	x	x		41	211
24	x	x	x	x	x	xx		9	223
25	x	x	x	x	x			20	231
26	x	x	x		x	x		17	241
27	x		x	x	x			17	249
28	x	x	x		xx	xx	xx	30	257
29	x	x	x		xx			17	267
30	x	x	x	x	xx			16	275
31	x	x	x	xxx	x			25	285
32	x	x	x	x	x	x		16	295

CHAPTER

1

Situational Assessment

In this chapter, the nurse manager is provided with a comprehensive list of resources from which to gain the data base necessary to promote effective nursing management. Distribution to students of the following outline would provide them a readily accessible check list for gathering the data they need to be effective nurse managers.

KEY TERMS

accreditation
beliefs
clientele
employee benefits
leadership style
licensure
litigation
management process
open system
primary care
professional nurse
registration
situational assessment
values

OUTLINE

I. Management process overview
  A. Definition
  B. Steps

II. Systems approach to situational assessment
  A. Three assessment areas for data gathering
    1. Work responsibilities
    2. Work environment
    3. Work force
  B. Use of systems approach in situational assessment
    1. Inputs
    2. Throughputs
    3. Outputs

III. Values and beliefs
  A. Past and present health care foci
  B. Application of societal values

IV. Organizational culture
  A. Values and beliefs
  B. Identification of guiding management principle
  C. Clinical or managerial value practices
  D. Agency history and role
    1. Influence upon services
    2. Guidance for future services

V. Agency governing board
  A. Responsibilities
    1. Legal role
    2. Functional role

- B. Nursing administrator's responsibilities
  - 1. Communication with board
  - 2. Meeting attendance
  - 3. Knowledge of board members

VI. Agency administrative personnel
- A. Knowing administrative personnel
  - 1. Educational and employment backgrounds
  - 2. Relationship background
  - 3. Philosophy
  - 4. Leadership style
- B. Organizational structure
  - 1. Formal
  - 2. Informal
  - 3. Centralization:decentralization
  - 4. Depth and breadth of organization
  - 5. Point of management decisions
  - 6. Liaison personnel
  - 7. Point of authority
- C. Leadership style
  - 1. Identification of role model
  - 2. Changing structures and impact

VII. Licensing and accreditation
- A. Licensing
- B. Licensing of nurses
  - 1. Definition of registration
    - a. Physician delegated exception
    - b. Revocation of licensure
  - 2. Role of nursing licensure
  - 3. Expanded role of the nurse
    - a. Professional nursing defined
    - b. Nurse practitioner regulations
- C. Licensing hospitals
  - 1. Role of state health departments
- D. Accreditation criteria for health agencies
  - 1. Role of Joint Commission on Accreditation of Healthcare Organization (JCAHO)
  - 2. Examples of JCAHO standards

VIII. Survey reports
- A. Review of reports
- B. Identification and correction of deficiencies

IX. Agency clientele
- A. Demographic data
- B. Geographical data
- C. Agency documents
- D. Health care user patterns

X. Agency services
- A. Types
- B. Scope
- C. Levels of primary care
- D. Employee oriented
- E. Rehabilitation

XI. Records
- A. Documentation method
- B. Documentation content

XII. Research
- A. Role of research
- B. Funding of research
- C. Oversight of research
- D. Current research

XIII. Educational programs
- A. Facility offerings
  - 1. Content and purpose of program
  - 2. Services to outside facilities
- B. Community offerings
  - 1. Community education programs
  - 2. Nursing organization programs

XIV. Salaries and fringe benefits
- A. Comparability with other health agencies
- B. Scope and nature of benefits

XV. Power structure
- A. Power defined
- B. Analysis of formal organizational structure
- C. Informal power structure
- D. Bureaucracy:adhocracy compared
- E. Power of position
- F. Power resistance tactics

XVI. Staffing
- A. Budgeted positions
- B. Job descriptions
- C. Role portrayal
  - 1. Nonverbal characteristics
  - 2. Verbal patterns
  - 3. Office milieu
- D. Differentiation and specification
  - 1. Examples
  - 2. Role confusion
  - 3. Role consistency
- E. Vice-President of Nursing
  - 1. Educational preparation
  - 2. Role in policy
  - 3. Salary comparisons
- F. Expansion of the nursing role
  - 1. Use of expanded roles
  - 2. Sources of conflict

G. Unit management system
H. Local labor pool
   1. Status of agency's labor pool
   2. Available options
   3. Community national labor trends
I. Nursing staff profiles
J. Staff licensure and certification status
   1. Verification of licensure
   2. Role of certification
K. Staff development
   1. State requirements
   2. Agency policies
   3. Continuing education program records

XVII. Communication techniques
A. Types of information
   1. Operational information
   2. Nonoperational information
B. Information systems
   1. Types
   2. Designated recipients
   3. Nature of input and output
C. Interpersonal communications

XVIII. Staff morale
A. Impact of organizational structure
B. Impact of and on change
C. Impact of communication lines

XIX. Work schedules
A. Types of
B. History of
C. Flexibility of
D. Centralized or decentralized responsibility

XX. Productivity measures
A. Current practices
B. Examples
C. Method

XXI. Union activity
A. Who is under union contracts
B. History of issues
C. Existing contracts
D. Preparing for negotiations
   1. Grievance history and process
   2. Current issues
   3. Union activities in area

XXII. Litigation
A. Sources of information
   1. Past and present litigation
      a. Nature of claims
      b. Nature of settlements
   2. Risk management committee
   3. Agency's legal officer
B. Preventive response examples

XXIII. Summary

OVERHEAD: Relationship of Nursing Process and Management Process

Nursing students at all levels are familiar with the nursing process. Comparison of the nursing process to the management process will provide meaningful transition into management thinking. Figure 1.1 at the end of this *Manual* may be copied and used as an overhead when presenting "I. Management process overview". (See outline above.)

CHAPTER OUTLINES

Distribution of chapter outlines to students can be supportive of student reading and/or class note taking. The first chapter may be most valuable (and less overwhelming) when presented as a survey chapter with the understanding that the content will be more fully developed in subsequent chapters. The use of the outline will provide a global viewpoint and aid in focusing student study.

Two different outline formats may be tried. Both provide support for either lectures or student reading/study.

Format 1: Present total outline on left half of page. Suggest that students take notes on the right side of page beside the concurrent outline topic.

Format 2: Reproduce outline leaving out key items for the student to fill in.

CLASS DISCUSSION: Community Healthcare Services

Time: 30 minutes

The nursing manager needs to be fully aware of health care services provided by her agency, and those provided by other agencies in the community.

- List the healthcare agencies in your community
- List the services provided by each agency.
  - Which services are duplicative and thus potentially competitive?
  - Which services require hi tech professionals?
  - Does the agency provide both "in-house" and "in-the-community" services?
  - What levels of care are provided?

GROUP DISCUSSION: Caring

Time: 30 minutes in small groups followed by discussion/summary time

Nursing students often react negatively to refocusing from "caring" perspectives to what is perceived as "business" perspectives. A positive climate for learning nursing management is promoted through this exercise.

Divide class into small groups.

Situation: Each group is to assume that they are a first level unit manager. In the role of first level manager what will they do to promote/facilitate the demonstration of caring among their nursing staff? (If there are several groups, one group can represent an acute care unit, another a long term care unit, another a home care supervisor, and another a medical clinic.)

GROUP ASSIGNMENT: Situational Assessment

Time: 30 minutes with follow up in next class.
Have each group give a ten minute report.

Situation: You are the new nurse manager in charge of outpatient services at ? hospital.

What information would you be wise to gather?
Where would you find the information?
Assign one of the following areas to each group:

1. Work responsibilities
2. Work environment
3. Work force

ASSIGNMENT: Values

Compare and contrast the values you see practiced with the values a health agency portrays in publicized media.

Criteria/focus might include:

identification of values
sources and content of publicized material
examples of practices which do or do not support the identified values
which practiced values are agency values
which practiced values counteract formalized agency values
recommendations derived from above

TEST QUESTIONS

KNOWLEDGE AND COMPREHENSION

True : False

T F 1.01. Health care agency values reflect changing cultural values.

T F 1.02. A nurse can expect health care agencies in the same community to practice the same values and beliefs.

T F 1.03. Knowledge of the organizational chart is adequate when seeking to learn communication channels.

T F 1.04. An effective nurse manager will seek to practice the same leadership style in all situations.

Multiple Choice

1.05. Good nursing management and problem solving utilize the scientific method. To practice a scientific method when problem solving, the nurse manager will first:
a. formulate a hypothesis or goal statement regarding the problem.
b. perform an audit of the problem area to identify the nature of the problem.
c. appoint an ad hoc committee to investigate the problem.
d. collect and/or compute relevant data to demonstrate the nature of the problem.

1.06. To acquaint him/herself with the position, the new nurse manager will want to conduct a situational assessment. This will best be done by:
a. attending an educational department orientation program
b. collecting information regarding the problem
c. prioritizing job responsibilities
d. collecting a wide scope of relevant agency information

1.07. The nurse manager practicing situational assessment within a systems approach will assess three broad areas as they relate to her position or tasks at hand. These areas are:
a. medical records, physician practices, patient case mix
b. staffing mix, patient case mix, patient records
c. staffing, organizational structure, services provided by agency
d. work to be done, working environment, staff

1.08. "Knowing" the agency administrator includes:
a. observing leadership style(s)
b. establishing a social relationship
c. learning of educational and employment background
d. a and c only
e. all of above

1.09. A manager can supervise ? employees if the employees perform fairly routine, similar tasks.
a. 5 or less
b. 10 to 20
c. 25 to 30
d. none of the above

1.10. A long-term care facility where decision making rests with the administrator is most likely to be described as a/an:
a. bureaucratic organization
b. matrix organization
c. adhocracy
d. decentralized organization

1.11. The new nurse manager should be knowledgeable about which of the following?
a. the state practice act
b. the agency licensing act
c. the medical practice act
d. a and c only
e. all of above

1.12. Which of the following best represents the purpose of licensure?
a. documents that minimum qualifications have been met
b. promotes a high quality standard of practice
c. enables an individual to use a particular title
d. a and c only
e. all of above

1.13. The agency responsible for licensing hospitals is:
a. JCAHO
b. state health department
c. county board
d. state medical board

1.14. Which of the following are true of the Joint Commission on Accreditation of Healthcare Organizations (JCAHO)?
a. has developed nursing standards
b. is a mandatory process
c. is a nongovernmental agency
d. a and c
e. all of above

1.15. In an adhocracy organization, job descriptions will be:
a. well defined
b. constantly evolving
c. unchanging
d. followed with care

1.16. The purpose of a unit management system is to:
a. relieve professional nurses of non-nursing functions
b. allow the nurse manager authority over all aspects of unit function
c. extend agency administrative influence into the unit level
d. a and c only
d. all of above

1.17. Which of the following is non-operational information needed by top and mid-level administration?
a. patient census data
b. monthly employee turnover rate
c. critical incident reports
d. patient classification data

1.18. Which of the following statements regarding employee morale is *true*.
a. Employee satisfaction is greater in organizations having clearly defined rigid role structuring.
b. Satisfied, committed employees are generally receptive to change.
c. Pressure to upgrade qualifications promotes staff morale.
d. Communication lines have little influence on staff morale.

APPLICATION, ANALYSIS, AND/OR SYNTHESIS

Multiple Choice

1.19. The agency board meeting schedule has been published. The nurse administrator should:
a. plan to attend
b. note the schedule and ask administrator for a report of relevant information
c. prepare and present updated nursing services information and goals
d. present written report to administration for presentation to board

1.20. As a new nurse manager of the outpatient unit you want to propose a new service. To support the program proposal you will:
a. survey potential users of the service
b. note agency's community contributions
c. portray the positive impact the service will have on agency image
d. a and c only
e. all of above

1.21. The nurse administrator observes that unit manager morale is lower following distribution of monthly computer generated status reports. Which of the following actions would most likely lead to improved morale?
a. do not give the unit managers the monthly status reports
b. meet with the unit managers and share the value of the reports
c. distribute select information from the monthly status reports
d. recommend that unit managers attend a staff support group

1.22. New nurse manager Ms. Wise wants to learn the power structure(s) influencing her position. Which of the following would be appropriate activities in which she should engage?
a. study the agency organizational chart
b. make sociogram at committee meetings and in the cafeteria
c. note communication link channels
d. all of above

1.23. Ms Wise asks Nurse Myownway to review discharge procedures and propose changes that will improve the negative patient feedback regarding discharge. Nurse Myownway agrees there is a problem but does not follow through. It is likely that Nurse Myownmway:
a. is resisting the power of Ms. Wise
b. likes to make patients dissatisfied
c. thinks that current procedures are just fine
d. a and c only
e. all of above

1.24. Nurse Manager Wise is preparing for contract negotiations. Ms. Wise will be wise to do which of the following?
a. compare salaries and benefits for the same workers in other agencies
b. note topics of recent grievances and their settlements
c. compare criteria for salary increments with other agencies
d. a and c only
e. all of above

1.25. Which of the following would be likely assumptions?
a. Nursing is expected to oversee the dietary and housekeeping departments.
b. The nursing administrator will supervise home care services.
c. Nursing power will be challenged.
d. all of above

1.26. Nurse Manager Wise would like to try several atypical scheduling options. In which of the following situations would she most likely be successful?
a. CICU abandoned 12 hour weekend shifts last year
b. outpatient O.R. needs to extend the operating schedule
c. pediatrics staff nurses have either been floated to other units or asked to take unpaid absence days
d. Nurse Manager Wise devises a plan for scattered shifts for the surgical floor to implement

ANSWERS		TEXT REFERENCE
1.01.	T	p. 10
1.02.	F	p. 12
1.03.	F	p. 14
1.04.	F	p. 16
1.05.	a	p. 9
1.06.	d	p. 9, 10
1.07.	d	p. 9
1.08.	d	p. 14
1.09.	b	p. 14
1.10.	a	p. 14, 15
1.11.	e	p. 16
1.12	d	p. 16
1.13.	b	p. 18
1.14.	d	p. 18
1.15.	b	p. 23
1.16.	d	p. 25
1.17.	b	p. 27
1.18.	b	p. 28
1.19.	c	p. 13
1.20.	e	p. 12, 13
1.21.	c	p. 14, 15
1.22.	d	p. 22, 23
1.23.	a	p. 23
1.24.	e	p. 29, 30
1.25.	c	p. 22
1.26.	b	p. 28, 29

CHAPTER

2

Management Theory

The second step of the management process is planning. The management theorists and theories presented in this chapter provide a foundation upon which nurse managers can base their planning.

KEY TERMS

administrative man
bureaucracy
economic man
quality circle
refreezing
satisficing
scientific management theory
system 4
theory x
theory y
theory z
unfreezing

OUTLINE

I. Historical background

II. Scholars and theorists
  A. Frederick Taylor
    1. Developed Scientific Management
      a. Based on research
      b. Time and motion studies
  B. Henri Fayol
    1. Identified management principles
    2. Promoted selection of principles to match situation
  C. Max Weber
    1. Advocated bureaucratic organizational structure
    2. Promoted specification of employee rights and duties
  D. Mary Follett
    1. Viewed management as a social process
    2. Suggested manager-employee exchange
  E. Elton Mayo and Fritz Roethlisberger
    1. Implemented Scientific Management theory
    2. Discovered Hawthorne effect
  F. Kurt Lewin
    1. Developed Field Theory of Human Behavior
      a. Identified phases of change: unfreezing, changing, refreezing

- G. Douglas MacGregor
  1. Explicated Theory X and Theory Y
     - a. Theory X views worker negatively in relation to work
     - b. Theory Y views worker positively in relation to work
- H. Chris Argyris
  1. Presented a maturational thesis
- I. Rensis Likert
  1. Advocated "System 4"
     - a. Emphasized democratic processes
     - b. Based on mutual trust
- J. Herbert Simon
  1. Differentiated between Economic Man and Administrative Man
  2. Stated steps of decision making
  3. Elaborated upon rational decision making
- K. Alvin Toffler
  1. Emphasized Future Shock
     - a. Impact of change
     - b. Need to guide, control, pace change
- L. Henry Mintzberg
  1. Challenged manager use of management process
  2. Identified ten managerial roles
     - a. Three interpersonal roles
     - b. Three informational roles
     - c. Four decisional roles
  3. Suggested managerial practice changes

III. Japanese management
- A. Comparison of Japanese and American management outcomes
- B. Japanese philosophy
  1. Concepts
  2. Influence of culture
  3. Employee advantages
  4. Hiring and educating practices
  5. Employee:company identification
- C. Theory "Z"
  1. Combines American and Japanese management practices
  2. Foci of Theory "Z"
  3. Quality circles
     - a. Defined
     - b. Purpose
     - c. Example
- D. Management principles of Yoshida

IV. Summary

DISCUSSION IDEAS

Chapter 2 objectives 1, 2, 6, and 7 may readily be used for class discussion.

GROUP ACTIVITY: Theories in Practice Setting

This group activity incorporates chapter objectives 2, 4, and 5.

Divide the class into small groups.

Time: 30 minutes for groups followed by discussion/summary time.

Group responses may be put on an overhead transparency and discussed with the entire class.

Situation: Each group is to assume that they are an individual looking for a first-level nursing management position. Two such positions are available in the community. One position is in a large physician's clinic; the other position is in a long-term care facility. The physician's clinic practices a management philosophy based upon Max Weber's and Frederick Taylor's theories and views the staff as functioning according to Theory X. The long-term care facility has an eclectic organizational orientation which incorporates aspects of Theory Y, Rensis Likert's, and Herbert Simon's perspectives.

Each group is to:

1. List the management orientation of each agency.

2. Based upon the management orientation, at which agency would you prefer to apply? Why?

Responses may include:
Clinic:
- bureaucratic organizational structure
- structured duties
- emphasis on productivity
- specified employee rights
- view of employee as lazy, more interested in paycheck than patients

Long-term care facility:
- practice of democratic management processes
- decentralized decision making
- mutual trust practiced
- view of employees as positive assets

ASSIGNMENT: Quality Circles

As a nurse administrator you would like to establish a quality circle.

1. In one paragraph:
   a. describe organizational characteristics which would facilitate the success of a quality circle, and
   b. which organizational characteristics would impede the success of a quality circle?
2. Write a two or three sentence "charge" for the quality circle. (A charge states the reason for the existence of a group and what the group is to accomplish.)

Comment: Some students find writing limits difficult. Learning to write succinctly is a coveted managerial skill. Exercises like this will help students develop such skills.

Responses:
1. a. Descriptions of an open decentralized organization with inclusion of select Japanese management practices are appropriate.
   b. Descriptions of bureaucratic organizational behaviors are expected.
2. Page 44 of the text states the purposes of quality circles: "(1) to engage employees in continuous planning evaluation, and improvement of work, materials and processes; and (2) to remove communication barriers between management and workers through frequent close interaction".

ASSIGNMENT: Theories in Practice

The assignment is most suitable for employed RN to BSN or graduate students.

Give two examples of management practices in an agency with which you are familiar.

For each example:
1. State the management theory/principle that is being followed;
2. compare and/or contrast the practice with Japanese management practices;
3. compare and/or contrast the practice with Theory Z.
4. For each example, state the management theory/principle you would recommend. State rationale for choice.

TEST QUESTIONS

KNOWLEDGE AND COMPREHENSION

True : False

T F 2.01. Theory X views employees positively.

Multiple Choice

2.02. Herbert Simon's Administrative Man makes rational decisions based upon:
- a. consideration of all alternative strategies.
- b. determining the consequences of each alternative.
- c. comparing evaluations of the consequences.
- d. all of above.
- e. none of the above.

2.03. Max Weber advocated a bureaucratic form of organization as one which would:
- a. promote creativity.
- b. be based on research.
- c. capitalize on employee maturational potential.
- d. provide a well-defined line of authority.

2.04. Which one of the following assumptions does *NOT* belong to McGregor's Theory Y?
- a. The average person learns, under proper conditions, both to seek and to accept responsibility.
- b. The expenditure of physical and mental effort in work is as natural as rest or play.
- c. The average individual prefers to be directed, hopes to avoid responsibility, and is more interested in financial incentives than in personal achievement.
- d. Man will exercise self-control and self-direction in the service of objectives to which he is personally committed.

2.05. To improve employee ability to cope with change, Toffler advocates that:
- a. employees perform time and motion studies to delete unnecessary activity.
- b. managers practice four decisional roles.
- c. employee maturational needs be considered by managers.
- d. that employees control their manner of response.

MATCHING: Match the theorist/scholar to the theory/principle s/he espouses by placing the appropriate letter in the space provided.

Theory/Management Principle

___ 2.06. scientific management would stimulate productivity

___ 2.07. used time and motions studies

___ 2.08. amount of authority and responsibility should match

___ 2.09. work should be divided and task specialization developed

___ 2.10. advocated bureaucracy as ideal structure

___ 2.11. saw management as a social process aimed at motivating employees to work toward a common end

___ 2.12. factors other than environmental conditions have greatest influence on worker productivity

___ 2.13. identified behavior change as unfreezing, changing, refreezing

___ 2.14. views workers positively and espouses participative management

___ 2.15. advocated a system of mutual employee/administrative trust

___ 2.16. concluded most managers make decisions that are good enough to fit minimum criteria

___ 2.17. combines Japanese and Ameri can management practices

Theorist/Scholar

a. Henri Fayol

b. Mary Follett

c. Kurt Lewin

d. Likert

e. Mayo and Roethlisberger

f. Mc Gregor

g. W. Ouchi

h. H. Simon

i. F. Taylor

j. Max Weber

APPLICATION, ANALYSIS, AND/OR SYNTHESIS

Multiple Choice

2.18. A consultant is hired to set up a process for costing nursing services. As an early step in the process, nurses are asked to keep an activity log of their time. The consultant is practicing which theory?

a. Frederick Taylor's time and motion studies.
b. Mayo's and Roethlisberger's Hawthorne effect.
c. Kurt Lewin's unfreezing step.
d. Mintzberg's role of liaison.

ANSWERS		TEXT REFERENCE
2.01.	F	p. 39
2.02.	e	p. 40

Rationale: the answer is "e" because Simon believes that today's manager cannot know all options and consequences, and must, therefore, choose the best from what is known. The work "satisficing" is used when discussing the manager's use of what is known as being good enough to act upon.

ANSWERS		TEXT REFERENCE
2.03.	d	p. 37
2.04.	c	p. 39
2.05.	d	p. 41
2.06.	i	p. 36
2.07.	i	p. 36
2.08.	a	p. 37
2.09.	a	p. 37
2.10.	j	p. 37
2.11.	b	p. 38
2.12.	e	p. 38
2.13.	c	p. 38, 39
2.14.	f	p. 39
2.15.	d	p. 36, 40
2.16.	h	p. 40
2.17.	g	p. 44
2.18.	a	p. 36

CHAPTER

3

Mission, Philosophy, Goals, Objectives

Students new to nursing management characteristically undervalue an agency's mission and philosophy statements. Through the study of the material presented in this chapter, students will see the usefulness and impact of carefully constructed agency mission and philosophy statements. The challenge for nurse managers is to see that the agency mission and philosophy are carried out through the goals and objectives of nursing. The activities presented below will aid students in valuing agency mission, philosophy, goal and objectives and their impact upon nursing practice.

KEY TERMS

conceptual framework
MBO
mission
objectives
philosophy
strategic planning

OUTLINE

I. Sequential organizational planning
  A. Agency mission
  B. Agency beliefs
  C. Relationship of nursing department conceptual framework, philosophy, mission to agency mission and beliefs
    1. Examples
    2. Content
      a. Person
      b. Environment
      c. Life
      d. Health
      e. Illness
      f. Nurse - patient relationship
      g. Nursing care
    3. Unit application and concurrence
  D. Short-term planning to accommodate change
  E. Foci of strategic planning
    1. Environmental threats and opportunities
    2. Structural strengths and weaknesses
  F. Planning direction

II. Management by objectives (MBO)
  A. Definition of MBO
  B. Purpose of MBO
  C. Effects of MBO
    1. Promotes interdependence of all levels

2. Improves worker self-esteem and self-actualization
3. Enhances worker self-esteem and self-actualization
4. Matures workers more rapidly
5. Promotes organizational efficiency
6. Promotes employee autonomy
7. Promotes organizational change

D. Advantages of MBO
1. Clarifies relationships and responsibilities of managers
2. Encourages delegation of responsibilities to subordinates
3. Promotes effective planning at all levels
4. Improves team and individual productivity
5. Improves worker morale
6. Promotes fair worker evaluations

E. Preparing staff for MBO
1. Brief employees on MBO
2. Share current nursing department purpose, objectives, and performance standards
3. Identify departmental stage of development
4. Periodically review progress
5. Formulate goals
6. Identify needs to attain goals seven questions to ask
7. Identify internal and external influencing factors
8. Update job descriptions

III. Preparing job objectives
A. Sample objectives for first-level nursing managers
B. Seven guidelines for formulating objectives
C. Negotiating objectives
1. Supervisor and employee design action plan
2. Establish time lines for review of progress

IV. Disadvantages of MBO
A. Limits focus to chosen objectives
B. Impedes managerial development
C. Permits neglect of "housekeeping" tasks
D. Focuses on outcomes while neglecting cost efficiencies
E. Allows unrecognized employee potential to remain unrecognized

V. Summary

OVERHEAD

Figure 3.1 at the end of the *Manual* may be used to present the relationships of the nursing conceptual framework, nursing philosophy, nursing mission, and nursing objectives.

DISCUSSION IDEAS

Identify a facility with which the group is familiar.

What conceptual framework provides the foundation for nursing practice?

How do you see the conceptual framework incorporated into nursing practice?

The above questions may also be applied to mission, philosophy, and objectives.

GROUP PROJECT: Mission Statements in Practice

(May be used as a homework assignment.)

Situation: You are a committee of nurses assigned the task of reviewing facility services and policies with the purpose of making recommendation that will better support the mission statement of the agency.

The mission statement of the agency includes:

a. providing quality cost effective health care for the service area
b. promote staff health and professional growth
c. promote community health

Have students divide themselves into groups of 3 - 5 students.

ASSIGNMENT A

1. Recommend services which would better reach out to serve the entire service area.
2. Write a policy which would support the second mission statement.
3. Make a recommendation regarding nurse staffing that would support the third mission statement.

Ideas for Assignment A responses:

1. The foci of the first mission statement are: quality care, cost effective care, and services to the service area. Students may focus on any one of these areas.
2. Policy supporting the second mission statement could focus on employee health or professional growth. For example, a policy recom mending a home visit and health assessment be made by the agency's home health care nurse on an employee's third sequential absent day.
3. Designating the use of "x" percentage of time of a well qualified specific staff position for community service development, implementation and follow up could stimulate positive outcomes.

ASSIGNMENT B

1. State a practice you see in a facility in your area which does not support the first mission statement.
2. Identify a policy which inhibits the practice of the second mission statement.
3. Identify a needed service that would support the third mission state ment.

GROUP ACTIVITY: Job Objective

This group activity incorporates chapter objectives 1 and 2.

Divide class into small groups.

Time: 30 - 45 minutes for writing objective followed by discussion/ summary.

Each group may write their objective on an overhead transparency and discuss how the resources listed below were incorporated in the writing of the objective.

Situation: You are in your second year of employment as a first-level nursing manager of an outpatient rehabilitation unit. Write one objective you will achieve in the coming nine months. Note how the objective relates to 1, 2, and 3 below.

Resources to use in writing objective:
What background information do you first need to know? Note Figure 3.1 in Manual. You may use the sample mission and philosophy statements presented on page 49 of text.

TEST QUESTIONS

KNOWLEDGE AND COMPREHENSION

True : False

T F 3.01. The writing of nursing objectives isthe first step in planning.

T F 3.02. Today the nurse manager needs to focus on long-range planning to best adjust to rapid changes.

T F 3.03. MBO improves worker productivity.

Multiple Choice

3.04. Organizational planning is a type of managerial decision making that includes:
1. investigating the environment
2. clarifying organization mission and philosophy
3. assessing organization resources
4. predicting effectiveness of alternative courses of action

a. 1, 2, 3
b. 1, 2, 4
c. 2, 3, 4
d. all of above

3.05. Strategic planning includes:
1. formulating a scheme of balancing scarce resources to achieve desired goals.
2. having a five year plan from which to operate.
3. assessment of environmental threats and opportunities.
4. clarifying agency mission and goals.

a. 1, 2, 3
b. 1, 3, 4
c. 2, 3, 4
d. all of above
e. none of above

3.06. A statement of nursing beliefs should include beliefs about the nature of:
1. health, illness
2. environment
3. life
4. nursing care

a. 1, 2, 3
b. 1, 2, 4
c. 2, 3, 4
d. all of above
e. none of above

3.07. Environmental assessment should include:
a. population shifts
b. changing health care patterns
c. competing agencies
d. all of above

3.08. Management by objectives promotes:
a. creativity.
b. useful long term planning.
c. focus on work outcomes.
d. quality control of everyday tasks.

3.09. At the heart of MBO is:
a. goal setting
b. decentralization
c. long term strategic planning
d. all of above

APPLICATION, ANALYSIS, AND/OR SYNTHESIS

Multiple Choice

3.10. The nurse manager was instructed by administration to institute MBO on her unit. She does not believe in MBO but conformed to the initial procedures she was to follow. Which of the following is most likely to occur?

a. staff were motivated to construct more productive goals
b. staff prioritized work according to the nurse manager's preferences
c. staff grew through the MBO process
d. all of above
e. none of above

3.11. The agency is practicing management by objectives. The unit head nurses are to present annual unit objectives to their staff at the next unit meeting. Implementation of the objectives is likely to have which of the following outcomes?

1. increased head nurse esteem
2. managerial growth in head nurses
3. head nurses focus on the stated objectives at the sacrifice of other needs areas
4. limited creative problem solving

a. 1, 2
b. 3, 4
c. 1, 2, 3
d. all of above
e. none of above

3.12. You as a nursing department head want to institute management by objectives (MBO) in your department. In what order will you see that the following are accomplished?

1. identify departmental stage of development.
2. update department purpose, objectives, and performance standards and share with employees.
3. implement objectives.
4. formulation of objectives by employees.
5. brief employees on MBO.
6. you and employee(s) negotiate objectives.

a. 5, 2, 1, 4, 6, 3
b. 4, 3, 6, 2, 1, 5
c. 6, 2, 4, 1, 5, 3
d. 3, 5, 1, 4, 6, 2

3.13. You are starting a new home care service. In which *order* will you develop the following?

1. objectives
2. philosophy
3. conceptual framework
4. mission

a. 1, 2, 3, 4
b. 2, 3, 1, 4
c. 3, 2, 4, 1
d. 4, 2, 3, 1

ANSWERS		TEXT REFERENCE
3.01.	F	p. 48
3.02.	F	p. 51
3.03.	T	p. 52
3.04.	d	p. 48
3.05.	b	p. 50, 51
3.06.	d	p. 49, 50
3.07.	d	p. 51
3.08.	c	p. 52
3.09.	a	p. 54
3.10.	e	p. 52
3.11.	d	p. 52, 53
3.12.	a	p. 54, 55
3.13.	c	p. 49

CHAPTER

4

Systems Approach

An understanding of systems theory will provide a framework in which the nurse manager can look at both the whole and the parts which make up the whole. The thirteen principles presented in the text (pages 73-75) and in Section XI of the outline below are particularly useful to the learner of systems theory. An *overhead* of Section XI of the following outline will help faculty to emphasize the importance of these principles when presenting the material.

KEY TERMS

closed system
deterministic system
dynamic system
feedback
input
open system
output
probabalistic system
static system
system
throughput

OUTLINE

I. Definition of systems approach

II. Characteristics of a system

III. Function of a system
  A. Rationale for systems approach

IV. Historical background
  A. Systems theorists
  B. Purpose and use

V. Significance to the nurse manager
  A. Examples of system types
  B. System uses
    1. Minimize negatives
    2. Maximize positives
    3. Analyze organizational functioning
    4. Prioritize resource use
    5. Decision making and problem solving tool
    6. Improve efficiency of work flow
    7. Evaluating effectiveness
    8. System outputs as outcomes
    9. Terminology as communication link

VI. Levels of system development
  A. Nine levels identified

VII. Classic system elements
  A. Role of seven elements of a system
  B. Relation of system to elements
  C. Definitions of system terms
    1. Environment
    2. Input
    3. Throughput

4. Output
5. Feedback and control

VIII. Subsystems
- A. Structure
- B. Interplay
- C. Required
- D. Personal
- E. Emergent

IX. Types of systems
- A. Natural and man-made
- B. Static and dynamic
- C. Deterministic and probabilistic
- D. Open and closed
- E. Centralized and decentralized
- F. External and internal
- G. Purposive and purposeful systems

X. Systems analysis
- A. Overview of use
- B. Techniques for system analysis
  1. Regression analysis
  2. Multiple regression analysis
  3. Model construction
  4. System simulation
  5. Linear programming
  6. Work sampling
  7. Work distribution charts
  8. Flow diagrams
  9. Forms analysis

XI. Basic systems principles
- A. Problem solving requires encompassing investigation
- B. System behaves in unique and characteristic manner
- C. Each system is also a subsystem
- D. System maintenance is central objective
- E. All systems are information systems
- F. Open system and its environment are highly interrelated
- G. Understanding of subsystems is essential to understanding the whole
- H. Relationships are of greater importance than objects to the system
- I. A change in one part of system changes all other parts
- J. When subsystems are in series, process alterations in any subsystem necessitate complementary alterations in related subsystems
- K. All systems tend toward equilibrium
- L. Changes in system boundary usually alter the function of certain subsystems and total system output
- M. To function smoothly a system must be strongly goal directed, must be governed by feedback, and must have the ability to adapt to changing external circumstances

XII. Introduction of new systems
- A. When needed
  1. Current system inadequate
  2. Development of new technology

XIII. Designing the system
- A. Overview
  1. Two approaches to take
  2. Five questions to ask
  3. Debugging of new system
- B. Principles of system design
  1. Nurse manager should work closely with system designer
  2. Role of each system component must be defined
  3. Feedback of each part is essential to output
  4. Specificity and intricacy of each system design should be adjusted to its purpose in the total system.
- C. Disadvantages of systems use
  1. Facilitates control of decision making
  2. Obscures complex relationships
  3. Fails to identify subtle power shifts
  4. Staff does not understand

XIV. Summary

CLASS ACTIVITY: Diagramming Subsystems

Time: 25 minutes

Ask students to imagine themselves as part of a home care service.

Faculty: Draw a large broken circle on the blackboard or overhead transparency to represent the home care service. The broken line of the circle represents a boundary through which exchange occurs.

QUESTIONS

1. Which systems principle does the broken circle representing a home care service portray?
   Answer: An open system and its environment are highly interrelated.

2. Does this broken circle represent an open or a closed system?
   Answer: Open system.

Ask students to identify components of a home care service.

Draw smaller circles within the larger circle and label the smaller circles as the identified components. Vary the sizes of the smaller circles.

Identify the smaller circles as subsystems of the home care service.

Once the larger circle is full, give a rationale for enlarging one of the subsystems. Demonstrate the difficulty of making room for the enlarged subsystem. Ask students for solutions.

QUESTIONS

3. Which systems principle does this represent?
   Answer: A change in one part of the system changes all other parts.

4. Does the above represent a static or a dynamic system?
   Answer: Dynamic

ASSIGNMENT: Diagram of System Interactions

Chapter objectives 1 and 2 may be used as a written assignment.

Objective 1:Diagram the budget system, the staffing system, or the quality-improvement system of your nursing organization, indicating several information, supply, and personnel inputs, throughput processes,product and service outputs, and principal feedback loops.

Objective 2: Indicate how the addition of another input, throughput process, or feedback loop could improve the function of the diagrammed system.

The assignment will be particularly useful for nurse managers and experienced RN to BSN students.

TEST QUESTIONS

KNOWLEDGE AND COMPREHENSION

True : False

T F 4.01. Systems theory can be applied to diverse scientific disciplines as well as to health care systems.

T F 4.02. A system is capable of maintaining some degree of organization in the midst of change.

T F 4.03. Systems analysis requires that the aspects being analyzed be fully quantified.

4.04. The elements of any system include goal,

a. input, throughput and output.
b. process and feedback.
c. control and environment.
d. all of above.

Matching: ***Match*** **the following entities with the system descriptor with which they relate.**

	Entities	System Descriptor
____	4.05. management process	a. closed system
____	4.06. nursing department	b. functional system
____	4.07. health agency	c. power system
		d. structural system

APPLICATION, ANALYSIS, AND/OR SYNTHESIS

True : False

T F 4.08. A health agency which views itself as a system will have continued existence as the central objective.

T F 4.09. A health care agency can function as a closed system in today's world.

Matching: As a nursing administrator of a health agency you may view the following as primarily serving which step in system function?

	System function	Steps
____	4.10. scheduling	a. input
____	4.11. policies	b. throughput
____	4.12. nursing assistants	c. output
____	4.13. nursing procedures	
____	4.14. patient care	

Matching: Match the term to the appropriate example by placing the letter in the space provided.

Example

____ 4.15. nursing care plan for Mr. Morris

____ 4.16. improved vital signs

____ 4.17. patient care process, staff development

____ 4.18. staff, supplies, budget, new governmental regulation, flooding

____ 4.19. research findings, quality improvement findings

____ 4.20. simulation, work sampling, model building

____ 4.21. nursing student who is developing greater expertise and self-confidence

____ 4.22. staff nurse refuses to use new equipment

____ 4.23. cardiac monitor set for 50-100 beats per minute

Terms

a. deterministic system

b. dynamic system

c. feedback

d. input

e. output

f. probabilistic system

g. static system

h. systems analysis

i. system's environment

j. throughput

Multiple Choice

4.24. The format for revising nursing practice standards in the coronary care unit includes "expected outcomes." The outcome information will provide:
a. input to nursing staff.
b. throughput to nursing auditors.
c. output for patient information.
d. all of above.

4.25. The revised nursing care standards now include expected outcomes. Which of the subsystems listed below will be impacted by the change?
1. direct care givers.
2. quality assurance reviewer.
3. patient.
4. administrative planners.
a. 1, 2
b. 2, 3
c. 1, 2, 3
d. all of above

ANSWERS		TEXT REFERENCE
4.01.	T	p. 61
4.02.	T	p. 60
4.03.	F	p. 72
4.04.	d	p. 65-67
4.05.	c	p. 62
4.06.	b	p. 62
4.07.	d	p. 62
4.08.	T	p. 70
4.09.	F	p. 70
4.10.	b	p. 66
4.11.	a	p. 66
4.12.	a	p. 66
4.13.	b	p. 66
4.14.	c	p. 67
4.15.	f	p. 70
4.16.	e	p. 67
4.17.	j	p. 66
4.18.	d	p. 66
4.19.	c	p. 67
4.20.	h	p. 63
4.21.	b	p. 69, 70
4.22.	g	p. 69
4.23.	a	p. 70
4.24.	d	p. 64
4.25.	d	p. 76, 77

CHAPTER

5

Budgeting

The nurse manager of today must become familiar with and participate in the planning, implementing and controlling aspects of budgeting. The various terms, tools, and processes introduced in this chapter will be useful as a communication link with accounting officers and administration. The practical theoretical base will help the budgeting novice and manager alike to make the budgeting process work for her/him and the services for which s/he is responsible.

KEY TERMS

allocation
breakeven point
budgeting
cost
cost accounting
decentralized budgeting
economic resources
financial control
fixed costs
H.M.O.
line item budget
operational budget
overhead
performance budgets
period costs
planning program
P.P.O.
real cost
roll-over budget
sunset budget
total cost
traditional budgets
unit of service
work sampling
zero based budgets

OUTLINE

I. Role and importance of nursing budgets
II. Historical background
   A. Budget types
      1. Traditional line item
         a. Characteristics
         b. Disadvantages
      2. Performance
         a. Response to Hoover commission
         b. Characteristics
         c. Disadvantages
      3. Planning program
      4. Zero-base
         a. History
         b. Defined
   B. Utilization review program
      1. Causes of cost crisis
      2. Responses to crisis

a. Managed care
b. Utilization review
c. Decentralizing budgeting

III. Purposes of budgeting
 A. Planning and controlling functions
 B. Primary purpose
 C. Secondary purposes
  1. Coordinating departments
  2. Orientation for managerial decisions
  3. Criterion for managerial performance
  4. Distinctive from cost accounting and cost reduction
  5. Communication of institutional priorities

IV. Definitions
 A. Economic resources
  1. Tangible assets
  2. Intangible assets
 B. Budgeting
  1. Definition
  2. Components
   a. Salaries
   b. Capital expenditures
   c. Operating expenses
 C. Related definitions
  1. Financial plan
  2. Operational budget
  3. Unit of service
  4. Program
  5. Financial control
  6. Allocation
 D. Costs and expenditures
  1. Costs
   a. Defined
   b. Real cost
   c. Total cost
  2. Types of costs
   a. Direct labor
   b. Indirect labor
   c. Fixed
   d. Semivariable
   e. Period
   f. Committed
   g. Programmed
   h. Overhead
  3. Capital expenditures
  4. Cost center
 E. Cost-benefit analysis
  1. Definition
  2. Breakeven point
 F. Accounting principles
  1. Conservatism
  2. Accrual

V. Types of budgets
 A. Components:
  1. Manpower
  2. Capital expenditure
  3. Operating
 B. Types
  1. Incremental
  2. Open-ended
  3. Fixed ceiling
  4. Flexible
  5. Roll-over
  6. Performance
  7. Program
  8. Zero-base
  9. Sunset

VI. Program budgeting
 A. Overview
 B. Value
 C. Advantages
  1. Managerial education
  2. Financial consequences
 D. Disadvantages
  1. Centralization of decision making
  2. Professional staff limitations

VII. Budgeting cycle
 A. Seven steps
 B. Examples
 C. Systems perspectives

VIII. Zero-base budgeting
 A. Nature
 B. Construction
  1. Decentralized
  2. Role of management levels
 C. Advantages
  1. Promotes managerial growth in fiscal accountability
  2. Controls costs
  3. Promotes objective fact finding
  4. Facilitates change
 D. Disadvantages
  1. Greater opportunity for communication failures
  2. Few operating managers are skilled in cost analysis
 E. Facilitating zero-base budgeting process
  1. Educate operating managers
  2. Establish budget phase time frames
  3. Develop/implement budget process procedures
  4. Provide relevant data

IX. Preparing for budgetary change
  A. Overview
    1. Prepare staff
      a. Instruction
      b. Manual
    2. Provide data
  B. Preparing the budget
    1. Develop decision package
    2. Preparing capital expenditure budget
    3. Preparing program budget
  C. Developing the nursing manpower budget
    1. Identify and evaluate alternatives
    2. Examples
    3. Sell merit of preferred option
  D. Direct nursing costs
    1. Identify standard cost target
    2. Manage by exception
    3. Problem identification
    4. Annual turnover rate
  E. Supply costs
  F. Flexible budget
    1. Defined
    2. Advantages
    3. Preparation considerations
  G. Tools used in budget preparation
    1. Work sampling
    2. Systems analysis
    3. Trend analysis
    4. Cost-benefit ratio
    5. Marginal analysis

X. Monitoring the budgeting process
  A. Overview
  B. Capital equipment and supply inventories
    1. Defined
    2. Supply/stock inventory lists
  C. Position control systems
    1. Need for system
    2. Use of serial number
  D. Supply control
  E. Financial reports
    1. Desired content
    2. Selective computer information
  F. Budget controls
    1. Need for system
    2. Needed rules/policies
  G. Problems in financial reporting
    1. Clarity
    2. Relevancy
    3. Balance
  H. Cost accounting
    1. Definition
    2. Responsibility accounting
      a. Definition
      b. Responsibility center
    3. Comparability
    4. Select data
    5. Examples
  I. Advantages of cost accounting
      a. Assess costs
      b. Identify interactions among cost items
      c. Identify hidden funding
  J. Disadvantages of cost accounting
      a. Identification of cost relationships
      b. Justifying costs with quantifiable outcome measures

XI. Variance analysis
  A. Defined
  B. Use in control
  C. Four step process
  D. Causative examples

XII. Summary

CLASS ACTIVITY: Budget Variance Report

The activity relates to chapter objective 4: "Identify, in a nursing unit's budget variance report, those areas of overspending that warrant immediate attention from the responsible nurse manager."

Time: 40 minutes

Activity:

Call the group's attention to Table 5.7, Sample Budget Variance Report, in the text.

Circle the items that have been *over*spent.

Underline the items that have been *under*spent.

Is the budget for this past month balanced, over, or under spent?

Answer: Individual items were overspent by $723.00, and underspent by $2323.80.
Total budget was underspent by $1600.80.

Considering these findings what would you as nurse manager do?

Discussion should include:

Did the decrease in regular personnel effect services? (Note savings which occurred through decrease use of regular personnel and small increase in registry personnel.)
Whether an increase in services occurred. (Note increased supply usages.)
Considering the underspending, were things not done that should have been done?

WRITTEN OR GROUP PROJECT: Cost Benefit Analysis

The focus of manpower costs in the exercise relate to chapter objectives 1 and 3.

Objective 1: Enumerate three major sections of the budget for a nursing unit, and describe three items included in each section.

Objective 3: Differentiate between direct and indirect labor costs, and specify one way to reduce each.

Faculty will want to go through the assignment with the entire class. As the items below are listed, the class can provide examples of what needs to be considered, e.g., what is to be included under direct and indirect staff costs.

Situation I: Podville Hospital is exploring the feasibility of a home IV therapy program. As a part of the proposal, you are to present at least two alternatives to a staffing approach with relevant cost-benefit analysis.

or

Situation II: Podville's long-term care facility is exploring the possibility of instituting a modular nursing staff model. Currently a functional nursing staff model is practiced on the unit which has 44 residents diagnosed as having Alzheimer's and/or behavioral needs. As a part of the proposal, you are to present at least two alternatives to a staffing approach with relevant cost-benefit analysis.

Identify:

percentage of reimbursement designated for manpower costs
type of staff needed
service unit
reimbursement per service unit
number of staff needed per number of service units
direct staff costs per position
indirect staff costs
breakeven point

Text pages 5-11 and 5-12 may be used as a reference.
Design alternative plans.
State which is the preferred alternative and why.

DISCUSSION IDEA: Budget types

Chapter objective 2 is useful as a quick chapter review at the beginning of the next class session.

Objective 2: Describe advantages and disadvantage of the following types of budget: line-item, performance, planning program, and zero based.

KNOWLEDGE AND COMPREHENSION

True : False

T F 5.01. The traditional line item budget is commonly used in health agencies today.

T F 5.02. The primary purpose of budgeting is to control dollar spending.

Multiple Choice

5.03. You are in a nursing management position. Which one of the following would best facilitate control?
- a. responsibility for budget.
- b. responsibility for hiring staff.
- c. responsibility for disciplining and firing staff.
- d. attending departmental meetings.

5.04. Which of the following contributed to the health care cost crisis?
1. increases in nursing salaries
2. hi tech equipment
3. consumer demand for wellness programs
4. overuse of complex diagnostic procedures

- a. 1,2,3
- b. 1,3,4
- c. 2,3,4
- d. all of above

5.05. Responses to increased health care costs include:
- a. managed care
- b. centralized budget planning
- c. low-tech options
- d. all of above

5.06. Which of the following are accurate statements when performing a cost-benefit analysis?
1. A ratio is calculated to demonstrate the relationship of costs to benefits.
2. The principle of conservatism is applied in keeping with accounting principles.
3. A breakeven point is identified.
4. All benefits must be reduced to monetary value.

- a. 1, 2, 3
- b. 2, 3, 4
- c. 1, 3, 4
- d. all of above

5.07. Cash flow problems arise out of the accrual system practice because:
- a. institutional payment for supplies is made at the time the consumer uses the supplies
- b. collected consumer payment is recorded as income.
- c. costs for supplies are charged when collected.
- d. income is recorded when services are rendered.

5.08. Which is characteristic of zero-base budgeting?
- a. based on budget of last year.
- b. decision making focuses on increases.
- c. speaks to growth mode.
- d. requires all expenditures to be reviewed.
- e. all of above.

5.09. Which of the following represents the function of variance reports?
a. aids in filling the controlling function of the budget.
b. compares actual spending to planned spending.
c. identifies spending trends.
d. all of above.

APPLICATION, ANALYSIS, AND/OR SYNTHESIS

Multiple Choice

5.10. Nursing administration practices decentralized budgeting. As nursing director which of the following types of budget would assist your first-level managers in downsizing?
a. traditional line item.
b. performance.
c. sunset.
d. zero-base.

5.11. As director of nursing in a nursing home which is experiencing an increase in acuity levels of patients, you plan to add an intense inservice program for nursing staff to update acute care nursing skills. Which of the following budget types would facilitate the costs involved with the inservice program?
a. traditional line item.
b. performance.
c. program.
d. flexible.

Matching: Match the budget section to the cost item by placing the letter in the space provided. You may use an answer more than once.

	Cost Item	Budget Section
____	5.12. purchase of land for parking	a. capital expenditure budget
____	5.13. nurse registry costs	b. manpower budget
____	5.14. cotton balls for nursing units	c. operating budget
____	5.15. consultant fees	
____	5.16. repair of sphygmomanometer	
____	5.17. computer terminals in patient rooms	

Matching: Match the answer from Column II to the item in Column I by placing the letter in the space provided. You may use an answer more than once. You may or may not use each answer.

	Column I	Column II
___	5.18. RN staff wages	a. capital expenditures
___	5.19. nursing administrator's salary	b. committed costs
___	5.20. 3-11 shift supervisor's salary	c. direct labor costs
___	5.21. liability insurance for nursing staff	d. indirect labor costs
___	5.22. institutional licensing fees	e. overhead
___	5.23. utilities	f. period costs
___	5.24. security patrol	g. programmed costs
___	5.25. new birthing chair	
___	5.26. nursing research	

Matching: Match the answer from Column II to the item in Column I by placing the letter in the space provided.

	Column I	Column II
___	5.27. Specified monies for a mammography screening program	a. allocation
___	5.28. Patient days, home visits, surgical procedures	b. cost center
___	5.29. Distribution of staff throughout facility	c. operational budget
___	5.30. All costs of mammography screening program	d. semivariable costs
___	5.31. Increase of inservice training hours for newly hired nurses	e. total costs
___	5.32. The pediatric inpatient unit	f. unit of service

Matching: Match the budget monitoring tool to the activity by placing the letter in the space provided. An answer may be used more than once.

Activity

____ 5.33. Listing furnishings in waiting room and staff lounge

____ 5.34. Listing of medications on all facility crash carts

____ 5.35. Statement of amount of designated FTE RNs used for out patient services

____ 5.36. Statement showing amount spent on sterile dressings and amount remaining for reporting period

____ 5.37. Statement showing cost of agency nurses exceeded budget

____ 5.38. Statement showing purchase of budgeted office supplies was not made

____ 5.39. Data listing total costs of new oral surgery outpatient treatment services

Budget Monitoring Tool

a. account reports

b. capital inventory

c. cost accounting

d. position control system

e. supply inventory

f. variance analysis

Matching: Match the budgeting tools to the activities by placing the letter in the space provided. You may use an answer more than once.

Activities

____ 5.40. Data showing new patient

____ 5.41. Data showing RN staffing patterns over last 3 years

____ 5.42. Data showing that additional staffing results in less output

____ 5.43. Data showing seasonal patterns of patient days

____ 5.44. Study of time required to perform a specific treatment

Budgeting Tools

a. cost-benefit ratio

b. marginal analysis

c. trend analysis

d. work sampling

ANSWERS		TEXT REFERENCE
5.01.	F	p. 83
5.02.	F	p. 84, 85
5.03.	a	p. 82, 83
5.04.	d	p. 84
5.05.	a	p. 84
5.06.	c	p. 87
5.07.	d	p. 87
5.08.	d	p. 84, 90-92
5.09.	d	p. 103-105
5.10.	b	p. 88
5.11.	c	p. 83, 84
5.12.	a	p. 86, 87
5.13.	b	p. 87
5.14.	c	p. 85
5.15.	b	p. 87
5.16.	c	p. 85
5.17.	a	p. 86, 87
5.18.	c	p. 86
5.19.	d	p. 86
5.20.	d	p. 86
5.21.	f	p. 86
5.22.	b	p. 86
5.23.	e	p. 86
5.24.	e	p. 86
5.25.	a	p. 86
5.26.	g	p. 86
5.27.	c	p. 85
5.28.	f	p. 85, 86
5.29.	a	p. 86
5.30.	e	p. 86
5.31	d	p. 86
5.32.	b	p. 86
5.33.	b	p. 99
5.34.	e	p. 99
5.35.	d	p. 99
5.36.	a	p. 101 (memo capsule)
5.37.	f	p. 103-105
5.38.	f	p. 103-105
5.39.	c	p. 102
5.40.	a	p. 87, 98
5.41.	c	p. 98
5.42.	b	p. 98
5.43.	c	p. 98
5.44.	d	p. 97

CHAPTER

6

Nursing Standards

Nursing standards contribute to the planning, implementing and controlling steps of the management process. The development and implementation of nursing standards follows system theory in the demonstration of input, throughput, and output. (See *Manual* Figure 6.1.) The more recent focus on outcome accountability has demonstrated the need for the development of relevant and timely nursing standards.

KEY WORDS

criterion
empirical standards
guideline
model
norm
normative standards
nursing care standard
nursing theory
objective
outcome standard
process standard
quality improvement
standard
structure standards

OUTLINE

I. Introduction

II. Definitions
- A. Standard
- B. Nursing care standard
- C. Guideline
- D. Objective
- E. Criterion
- F. Norm
- G. Model
- H. Patient problem
- I. Nursing problem
- J. Quality improvement
- K. Nursing orders
- L. Nursing audit

III. Purposes of nursing care standards
- A. Improve quality of nursing care
- B. Decrease cost of nursing care
- C. Provide bases for determining nursing negligence

IV. Sources of nursing care standards
- A. American Nurses' Association
  1. Standards of Care
  2. Standards of Professional Performance
- B. State and local nursing groups
- C. University nursing schools

V. Types of nursing care standards
   A. Normative or empirical
   B. Structure, process, or outcomes
   C. General or specific statements of expected quality
   D. Examples

VI. Organizing staff for standards writing
   A. Input
      1. Nursing philosophy and objectives
      2. Nursing priorities
      3. Nursing theory
      4. Identified needs
   B. Relationship of nursing theory to standards
      1. Theory identifies clients, goal, and interventions
      2. Examples applied
         a. Orem
         b. Rogers
         c. Roy
         d. Neuman
   C. Topics for standards development
      1. Choose normative or empirical approach
      2. Identifying need
      3. Use of Maslow's Hierarchy of Human Needs
         a. Categories
         b. Needs
      4. Guide for nursing activities
         a. Structure, process, outcome
         b. Examples
   D. Standards task force
      1. Composition
      2. Development process

VII. Legal significance of standards
   A. Malpractice
   B. Use of national standards

VIII. Revision of nursing care standards
   A. Use as working model
   B. Responsive to change

IX. Summary

OVERHEAD

Figure 6.1 at the end of this *Manual* may be used as an overhead to aid the student in applying system theory and the management process to the role of nursing standards.

GROUP ACTIVITY: Standards

Chapter objective 3 can readily be adapted as a group activity: "Write one example of a structure standard, one example of a process standard, and one example of an outcome standard that apply to nursing practice in your clinical nursing specialty." Designate whether the standard is a "normative" or an "empirical" standard.

Historically, the earlier nursing standards tended to be structure standards, then as nursing process became widely practiced, process standards were emphasized. As consumers, government and various agencies demanded to know the effectiveness of health care, outcome standards were developed. The nurse manager needs to be cognizant of all three types of standards and the value of each.

If the class is divided into three groups, one group can be assigned to write a structure standard, the second group a process standard, and the third group an outcome standard for a unit with which they are familiar. To reinforce management learning, the standard could focus on an aspect of management concern; i.e., staff development, quality improvement, safety.

TEST QUESTIONS

KNOWLEDGE AND COMPREHENSION

True : False

T F 6.01. Standards of nursing care will be comparable from one agency to another.

Multiple Choice

6.02. Which of the following are true of nursing standards? Standards:
1. are used to plan and control care.
2. contain desired outcomes.
3. provide a basis for determining nursing malpractice.
4. are basic to implementation of quality assurance.

a. 1, 2, 3
b. 2, 3, 4
c. 1, 2
d. all of above

6.03. Which of the following is true of a nursing norm?
a. represents the current level of actual nursing practice.
b. is a value-free description of an indicator of patient care quality.
c. is the process of establishing desirable standards of nursing practice.
d. makes a concrete statement of intention, or goal toward which effort is directed.
e. all of above.

6.04. The American Nurses' Association, state and local nursing organizations, and university nursing schools are all potential sources for:
a. quality assurance programs.
b. nursing standards.
c. identifying norms.
d. all of above.

6.05. You are to chair a standards review task force. What information will you provide to committee members in preparation for the first meeting?
a. nursing philosophy and nursing theory to be practiced
b. nursing priorities
c. list of areas of concern
d. all of above

Matching: Match the term to the definition by placing the letter in the space provided.

	Definition	Term
___	6.06. current level of performance	a. criterion
___	6.07. value-free description of a variable believed to be an indicator of patient care	b. guideline
___	6.08. a concrete statement of intention toward which effort is directed	c. norm
___	6.09. a recommended path to safe conduct	d. objective
___	6.10. an authoritative statement enunciated by a profession by which quality of practice, service, or education can be judged	e. standard

Matching: Match the type of standard to the appropriate characteristic by placing the letter in the space provided.

	Characteristic	Type of Standard
___	6.11. good or ideal	a. empirical
___	6.12. group or institution oriented	b. normative
___	6.13. methods for nursing care	c. outcome
___	6.14. observed practice in many	d. process
___	6.15. patient care results	e. structure

APPLICATION, ANALYSIS, AND/OR SYNTHESIS

Multiple Choice

6.16. You are manager of a home care service which has adapted *Orem's self care* theory. Which of the following demonstrates an *outcome* focus for which a nursing standard would be written?

a. The patient's acceptance of limited mobility.
b. The patient's compliance with medication regime.
c. The patient's level of coping with disease process.
d. The patient's method of obtaining proper nutrition.

6.17. You are a nurse in an area rehabilitation center which utilizes Roy's theory. Which of the following demonstrates a *process* focus for which a nursing standard would be written?

a. Promotion of client's adaptation to condition.
b. Level of paraplegics' mobility.
c. ADLs which clients can perform for themselves.
d. Ability to use outside resources for health and maintenance needs.

6.18. Nurse Jones is being sued for malpractice by a patient to whom she was assigned. Nurse Jones is confident that she will not be found guilty because she:

a. gave the patient the best care she could.
b. followed the care outlined by the nurse whom she relieved.
c. followed appropriate standards of care.
d. all of above.

ANSWERS		TEXT REFERENCE
6.01.	F	p. 107
6.02.	d	p. 108
6.03.	a	p. 108
6.04.	b	p. 109
6.05.	d	p. 112
6.06.	c	p. 108
6.07.	a	p. 107, 108
6.08.	d	p. 108
6.09.	b	p. 108
6.10.	e	p. 107
6.11.	b	p. 110
6.12.	e	p. 110
6.13.	d	p. 110
6.14.	a	p. 110
6.15.	c	p. 110
6.16.	b	p. 111, 113
6.17.	a	p. 113
6.18.	c	p. 116

CHAPTER

7

Organizational Structure

The many changes in the health care delivery system of recent years have forced health care agencies to restructure services, to downsize in some areas and add services in other areas and simultaneously assign greater accountability to each service area. This has led to restructuring of agencies and nursing departments, retitling positions and downward delegation of responsibilities and decision making. Current formal organizational diagrams can provide useful information about the emerging status and philosophy of nursing practice. Figures 7.1 and 7.2 in the back of this *Manual* and the accompanying discussion questions will help your students discover changes which reflect philosophy, authority and potential problems. Perhaps formal organizational structure has been somewhat neglected by nursing, but today is a vital part of defining what nursing is to be.

KEY TERMS

administrative model
authority
average organizational distance
centralization
coercive power
congressional model
councilor model
decentralization
expert power
formal structure
functionalized line and staff
hierarchy
informal structure
line and staff
line organization
matrix
referent power
relative organizational distance
reward power
shared governance
total organizational distance

OUTLINE

I. Formal and informal structure
   A. Overview
   B. Roles

II. Formal table of organization
   A. Motivation for change
   B. Diagramming organization structure
      1. Components identified
      2. Relationships demonstrated
      3. Significance of structure
   C. Uses for a formal table of organization
      1. Shows relationships of positions
      2. System of power and control
      3. Clarifies functions

III. Organization characteristics
   A. Span of control
      1. Supervisor:employee ratios
      2. Influencing factors
   B. Organizational principles

1. Unity of command
2. Requisite authority
3. Continuing responsibility
4. Organizational centrality
5. Principle of exceptions

C. Organizational concepts
1. Role
2. Power
   a. Definition
   b. Value
   c. Types
   d. Amount
3. Status
   a. Defined
   b. Relationship to rewards
   c. Relationship to resources
4. Responsibility
5. Authority
6. Centrality
   a. Total organizational distance
   b. Average organizational distance
   c. Relative organizational distance
7. Communication

D. Centralization versus decentralization
1. Definitions
2. Characteristics
3. Role of delegation
4. Impact on personnel

IV. Types of formal organization structures

A. Line organization
1. Background
2. Nature and role of staff
3. Functions of staff: service, advise, control
4. Advantages
5. Disadvantages

B. Line and staff organization
1. Defined
2. Functions of staff
3. Advantages
4. Disadvantages

C. Functionalized line and staff organization
1. Description
2. Advantages
3. Disadvantages

D. Matrix structure
1. General background
2. Ad hoc project teams
   a. Defined
   b. Use
   c. Impact
3. Organization
   a. Characteristics
   b. Impact
      (1) On job satisfaction
      (2) On relationships
      (3) On nursing administration
   c. Redefining authority, responsibility, and accountability
4. Five questions to clarify decision/action roles

E. Shared governance
1. Definitions
   a. Councilor model
   b. Congressional model
   c. Administrative model
2. Goal
3. Structure
4. Impact

V. Committees

A. Overview
1. Definition and role
2. Functions

B. Advantages and disadvantages

C. Ideal size

D. Three functional stages

VI. Organizational retrenchment

A. Need for

B. Computations for

C. Conduct of

VI. Summary

DISCUSSION IDEAS: Organizational Structure at Work

The following incorporates chapter objectives 1, 2, and 3.

Objective 1: Draw a diagram of the formal organizational structure of your nursing department.

Objective 2: Describe one advantage and one disadvantage of each of the following organizational structures: pure line, line and staff, functionalized line and staff, matrix, shared governance.

Objective 3: Explain the relationship between responsibility and authority under ideal circumstances.

Figures 7.1 and 7.2 (at the end of this *Manual*) are the basis upon which the discussion is developed. You will want to copy the figures for students or use overheads to present the figures.

1. Look at Figures 7.1 and 7.2. What type of organizational structure do these diagrams describe?

Answer: Line and staff. The quality assurance, utilization review and risk management areas provide support services to the hospital administrator. Nursing administration, too, uses supportive staff which can be found in the infection control and staffing positions.

2. Communication lines:

Activity: Ask students to draw communication lines promoted by the Podville nursing department organizational chart. (Figure 7.2 at back of the *Manual*.)

Questions:

a. What lines of communication are potentially problematic?

b. How could the clinical specialists communicate more effectively?

Possible responses:

a. Vertical communication lines are strong thus promoting authoritative downward communications and feedback upward communications. Competition rather than cooperation will also be promoted. Distance of infection control and project specialist personnel may dilute their direct influence on care delivery.
Consider the special patient services under the president. (See Figure 7.1.) Nursing has little or no communication with special patient services.

b. Clinical specialists do not directly communicate with care units and must go through multiple layers to get to special patient services.

3. The staff nurses for inpatient care forward few referrals to home care and hospice even though there are discharge patients who would profit from these services. Is the organizational structure at least partly responsible for the problem? How could the organizational structure be changed to support the use of home care and hospice services?

Analysis: More recent types of patient care services, home care, hospice, outpatient services, and perhaps occupational health, are directly responsible to the administrator. This may suggest one or all of the following:

a. the impetus for developing these services came from the administrator.

b. the administrator wants to closely monitor the new services.

c. the new services may be structured to be fiscally independent.

d. the nursing department did not embrace the responsibilities of these new services for any number of reasons.

Answer: The direct reporting to the administrator rather than to nursing administration isolates the services from other nursing staff. The placement of all nursing services under the nursing department would provide formal structural support for improved communication and interaction.

4. Note the vice president titles and their place in the organizational chart. If the titles and placement reflect institutional philosophies, how are nurses perceived?

Analysis: Note that all department head titles including nursing are prefaced with vice president; all are placed at the same level; all report to the administrator. Note also that the vice president titles are followed by a designation of the departmental area. A comparison should be noted at this point: one department is "professional services," another department is "nursing services."

Answer: Nursing is perceived as a department of equal importance to three other departments. Top nursing administration is accorded the same title as the three other department heads. However, the coexistence of a department of professional services as well as a department of nursing may reflect that nursing is viewed not as a professional service but rather as a technical service.

5. In Figure 7.2 you may note the clinical specialist positions.

a. What type of power do they have?

Answer: Expert power.

b. What would the expected relationship be between the Operating Room Director and the Director Medical/Surgical Nursing?

Answer: The chart communication lines show no direct connections. If formal lines are followed, the relationship would be quite distant.

TEST QUESTIONS

KNOWLEDGE AND COMPREHENSION

True : False

T F 7.01. An organization's formal structure limits and focusses communication between employees.

T F 7.02. An organizational structure should provide a wider span of control for the nurse executive than for first-level managers.

T F 7.03. The most important factor in determining a manager's optimum span of control is the number of subordinates.

T F 7.04. The amount of information given a worker affects the quality of his/her work.

Multiple Choice

7.05. Formal plus informal organizational structure determine:
- a. work flow and interpersonal relationships.
- b. budgetary allocations.
- c. planned communication avenues.
- d. quality assurance foci.

7.06. Which of the following are characteristics of formal organization structure?
1. based upon institutional philosophy, goals and objectives.
2. determines the amount and type of communication between staff members.
3. indicates the degree of authority of positions.
4. indicates span of control of positions.
- a. 1, 2, 3
- b. 2, 3, 4
- c. 1, 2, 4
- d. 1, 3, 4

7.07. When participative management is practiced, communication will be:
- a. downward
- b. upward
- c. lateral
- d. all of above

7.08. The nursing administrator is going to appoint a committee to explore improvement of discharge follow-up. To promote effective committee function how many persons will she appoint?
- a. 3.
- b. 4-5.
- c. 6-8.
- d. 10-12.

Matching: Match the items in Column II to Column I by placing the letter in the space provided.

	Column I	Column II
___	7.09. An employee should be responsible to only one supervisor	a. continuing responsibility
___	7.10. Control over resources	b. manage by exception
___	7.11. Supervise delegatee	c. organizational centrality
___	7.12. Information crosspoint	d. requisite authority
___	7.13. Scrutinize the unexpected	e. unity of command

Matching: Match the terms to the appropriate description by placing the letter in the space provided.

	Description	Terms
___	7.14. expected behaviors	a. authority
___	7.15. push/pull force	b. power
___	7.16. rank/recognition	c. responsibility
___	7.17. clout/sanction	d. role
___	7.18. obligation for one's conduct	e. status

Matching: Match the organization structure type to its characteristics by placing the appropriate letter in the space provided. Answers will be used more than once.

	Characteristics	Structural Type
____	7.19. weak integration of departments	a. line and staff
____	7.20. staff officers have some authority over line employees	b. line organization
		c. functionalized line and staff
____	7.21. continuous use of project teams confuses roles	d. matrix
____	7.22. free-form, shifting relationships	e. shared governance
____	7.23. goal is to increase nurses' autonomy and recognition	
____	7.24. support for executives	
____	7.25. authority confusion	
____	7.26. simple, rigid	
____	7.27. stimulates nurses to a high level of motivation	
____	7.28. nursing practice is controlled through collaboration	
____	7.29. specialists are coordinated both vertically and horizontally	
____	7.30. staff officers have less power than line officers	

APPLICATION, ANALYSIS, AND/OR SYNTHESIS

Multiple Choice

7.31. As a money saving measure, the hospital administrator issued a memo saying that the bedtime nourishments from the dietary department will be discontinued. In a line and staff organizational structure, which of the following actions should the nurse take?
a. Consult the dietary supervisor.
b. Form an ad hoc committee to put pressure on the hospital administrator.
c. Talk to the immediate supervisor.
d. Invite the patients' families to bring in food.

7.32. Which of these first level nursing position functions is characteristic of a decentralized management system?
1. Participating in interdisciplinary team meeting on the unit.
2. Submitting daily patient acuity level forms.
3. Determining the staffing pattern for nursing personnel for the unit.
4. Determining the unit budget.
5. Implement staff evaluation processes.
a. 1, 2, 3
b. 2, 3, 4
c. 2, 4, 5
d. all of above

7.33. You are a cardiac nurse specialist and desire a position which will allow you to use your high level of clinical cardiac expertise. Which organizational structure would theoretically best support you in utilizing your expertise?
a. adhocracy.
b. line.
c. line and staff.
d. functionalized.

7.34. As a cardiac nurse specialist, what type of power are you most likely to have?
a. expert
b. coercive
c. reward
d. referent

7.35. Which of the following situations best illustrates the principle of "Requisite Authority" in practice?
a. Head nurse D.O. Moor is asked by nursing administration to write a proposal for discharge patient follow-up.
b. The facility practices centralized staffing. Head Nurse N.A. Ivete receives a warning regarding excessive staffing costs.
c. Inservice Director I.M. Goodson allocates the inservice budget to support the scheduled programs.
d. Special services Director T.L. Metoo is instructed to implement the new service in the department.

7.36. Director Del Agate is to present a report in two weeks on the uses of specified services. She asked the first level manager to prepare an audit of the use of a service for the last six months. The report is not ready on time. Who is responsible for the tardy report?
a. Director Del Agate.
b. first level manager.
c. supervisor.
d. none of the above.

7.37. The above situation is an application of which principle?
a. unity of command.
b. continuing responsibility.
c. organizational centrality.
d. exceptions.

7.38. Nursing Administrator P.R. Ticipate values the expertise of various staff nurses and appoints nurses to many various committees which make recommendations that are usually accepted. What impact will this on-going management practice have on the formal organizational structure?
a. weaken the formal structure.
b. reinforce authority lines in the formal structure.
c. support the formal structure by providing needed expertise.
d. all of above.

ANSWERS	TEXT REFERENCE
7.01. T	p. 125
7.02. F	p. 125
7.03. F	p. 125
7.04. T	p. 129
7.05. a	p. 123, 124
7.06. c	p. 124
7.07. d	p. 130
7.08. c	p. 144
7.09. e	p. 126
7.10. d	p. 126
7.11. a	p. 126
7.12. c	p. 126
7.13. b	p. 126
7.14. d	p. 126, 129
7.15. b	p. 127, 129
7.16. e	p. 128, 129
7.17. a	p. 128, 129
7.18. c	p. 128, 129
7.19. b	p. 132-135
7.20. c	p. 137
7.21. d	p. 138
7.22. d	p. 138
7.23. e	p. 142, 143
7.24. a	p. 135-137
7.25. d	p. 138
7.26. b	p. 132-135
7.27. d	p. 138
7.28. e	p. 142, 143
7.29. d	p. 138
7.30. a	p. 135-137
7.31. c	p. 132
7.32. d	p. 131
7.33. d	p. 137
7.34. a	p. 127
7.35. c	p. 126
7.36. a	p. 126
7.37. b	p. 126
7.38. a	p. 134

CHAPTER

8

Job Analysis and Evaluation

Job analysis and evaluation are key to many administrative functions. The chapter supplies information and tools for job analyses necessary to the writing of useful job/position descriptions. Faculty may choose from the assignments and group activities, the exercises which best meet the level of student readiness.

KEY TERMS

benchmark job
career ladders
career mobility
compensable factors
field theory
job
job analysis
job classification
job description
job evaluation
job grade
job specifications
policy
position
procedure
salaries
task
wages
work sampling

OUTLINE

I. Introduction to job analysis and evalution
  A. Challenge
  B. Use

II. Wage and salary structure
  A. Need for fair salary structures
  B. Salary and employee expectations
  C. Relationship between pay and job satisfaction
    1. Theoretical perspectives
      a. Herzberg's dissatisfiers
      b. Lewin's field theory
      c. Jaques: C-W-P balance
    2. Problems arising from inequity in work-pay relationships

III. Career ladders and lattices
  A. Value of promotion from within

- B. Advantages of career ladders
- IV. Job evaluation process
  - A. Job evaluation
    1. Rationale
    2. Definition
    3. Purpose
  - B. Definitions
    1. Policy
    2. Procedure
    3. Wages
    4. Salaries
    5. Task
    6. Position
    7. Job
    8. Benchmark job
    9. Job grade or job classification
    10. Job analysis
    11. Job description
    12. Job specifications
  - C. Job evaluation committee
    1. Composition
    2. Process
  - D. Job analysis
    1. Duties and responsibilities
    2. Skills and personal attributes
    3. Factors to include
    4. Example
    5. Process
  - E. Collecting job information
    1. Content to be considered
       - a. Job oriented work activities
       - b. Employee oriented work behaviors
       - c. Machines, tools, and aids used
       - d. Knowledge used
       - e. Working conditions
       - f. Personal requirements
    2. Methods of collection
       - a. Questionnaire
       - b. Self-report diary
       - c. Interview
       - d. Observation
       - e. Work sampling
  - F. Compensable factors
    1. Defined
    2. Examples
  - G. Job description
    1. Definition
    2. Purposes
       - a. Job evaluation
       - b. Wage and salary administration
       - c. Manpower planning
       - d. Employee evaluation
       - e. Assist with recruitment, selection, orientation, recruitment and replacement
       - f. Legal documentation
    2. Construction
       - a. Sociotechnical
       - b. Standardized format
       - c. Content
         - (1). Title
         - (2). Summary statement
         - (3). Reporting relationships
         - (4). Job tasks
         - (5). Job resources
         - (6). Job context
         - (7). Job specifications
    3. Review of job description
       - a. Worker, supervisor
       - b. Compare with standard job description
       - c. Periodic review
  - H. Methods of job evaluation
    1. Job ranking
       - a. Defined
       - b. Method
       - c. Example given
       - d. Advantages and disadvantages
    2. Job classification
       - a. Job grades
       - b. Benchmark jobs
       - c. Grade example
    3. Factor comparison method
       - a. Definition
       - b. Process
       - c. Advantage and disadvantage
       - d. Evaluation
    4. Point system
       - a. Description
       - b. Implementation
       - c. Advantage
       - d. Process
  - I. Job redesign
    1. Job rotation
    2. Job enlargement
    3. Job enrichment
- V. Summary

ASSIGNMENT: Position Description

Chapter objectives 2 and 4 are met in this assignment.

Objective 2: Identify the component tasks included in your job description and estimate proportion of time devoted to each.

Objective 4: Rewrite your own job description to clarify component tasks and the amount of each compensable factor.

Activities

1. Obtain the most up-to-date description for the job/position you currently hold. (For generic BSN students faculty may provide a job description.)
2. Identify the written component tasks that are included in the job /position description.
3. Identify the component tasks that are included in job/position expectancies that are not written.
4. Identify the component tasks that should be included and are not. (Use ANA, JCAH, or other relevant standards to guide in the identification of these tasks.)
5. Utilizing the above information, rewrite the job/position description using the format presented in Figure 8.1 at the back of the *Manual.*
6. Add a column at the left of the position description and assign an approximate percentage of time to each responsibility.
7. Append the old job/position description.

ASSIGNMENT: Benchmark Job

Chapter objective 1 is met in this assignment: "Read the job descriptions for all nursing positions in your agency and identify a benchmark job against which to evaluate other nursing positions."

Activities

1. Review all nursing job descriptions.
2. Identify three job descriptions which represent a sizable percentage of the total nursing staff. State the approximate percentage and budgeted FTE for each of the job descriptions.
3. Of the identified job descriptions, which job description contains the most stable job content over time? Identify the stable items.

4. Is this job generally well known to nursing staff and nursing administrators?

   If yes, the job may be an appropriate choice to use as a bench mark job description.

   If no, consider the second and third job descriptions selected above for use as a bench mark job description.

   The addition of the following activity will meet chapter objective 3 to identify compensable factors.

5. Having identified the job description that is to become the bench mark job description, state the compensable factors that are present.

DISCUSSION: Compensable Factors

Objective 3 may be used as a class discussion topic: "Identify four compensable factors that are present in all jobs in your agency's nursing hierarchy".

GROUP ACTIVITY: Rank Order

Objective 5: "Rank the nursing jobs in your agency according to your perception of their complexity and difficulty".

Time: 30 minutes plus discussion time

Divide class into small groups.

Assignment

1. List the nursing jobs for Podville Hospital. Use Figures 7.1 and 7.2 at the back of te *Manual* when making list.
2. Rank order positions according to degree of complexity and difficulty.
3. List the factors you considered when ranking positions.

TEST QUESTIONS

KNOWLEDGE AND COMPREHENSION

True : False

T F 8.01. The use of "other tasks as assigned by___" is a desirable statement in a position description.

T F 8.02. A rank order system is better suited to job evaluation in a health agency because several job families are represented in the work force.

T F 8.03. According to the text, enlargement of a job increases job satisfaction.

Multiple Choice

8.04. Which of the following are appropriate uses of job descriptions?
1. sorting/recording job tasks.
2. facilitating wage and salary administration.
3. providing a basis for manpower planning.
4. assisting with recruitment, selection, placement, orientation and dismissal of employees.

a. 1, 2, 3
b. 1, 3, 4
c. 2, 3, 4
d. all of above

8.05. At what level will employee expectations and real salary discrepancies likely lead to employee open reaction? Salaries are:

a. + or - 1% of expectancy.
b. + or - 3% of expectancy.
c. + or - 5% of expectancy.
d. + or - 10% of expectancy.

8.06. A quality position description will contain which of the following?
1. minimum educational requirements
2. required credentials/licensure
3. activities/responsibilities of position
4. performance standards
5. stated salary

a. 1, 2, 3, 4
b. 2, 3, 4, 5
c. 1, 3, 5
d. all of above

8.07. The *first* steps in job evaluation are to:
1. determine the duties and responsibilities associated with the job.
2. determine the skills and personal attributes required for the job.
3. identify performance standards.
4. observe actual job performance of employee being evaluated.

a. 1, 2
b. 2, 3
c. 3, 4
d. 1, 4

8.08. The simplest, quickest, least precise means of job evaluation is:

a. job ranking
b. job grading
c. work sampling
d. job classification

Matching: Match the term to the definition by placing the letter in the space provided.

	Definitions	Terms
____	8.09. long-range statement of organizational objectives	a. job
____	8.10. statement of technique used to obtain goal	b. policy
____	8.11. a group of activities and responsibilities	c. position
____	8.12. work assignment	d. procedures
____	8.13. financial compensation for services rendered	e. task
____	8.14. a series of work activities for a purpose	f. wages

APPLICATION, ANALYSIS, AND/OR SYNTHESIS

Multiple Choice

8.15. In what order would you do the following when writing or revising a job description?
1. compare one job with another
2. compare position againt standard
3. group job tasks
4. have employee and supervisor critique job description
5. identify job resources
6. specify working conditions

a. 1, 2, 4, 3, 5, 6
b. 3, 5, 6, 1, 4, 2
c. 4, 5, 1, 3, 2, 6
d. 6, 3, 4, 5, 1, 2

8.16. Nurse manager Bee Ware is preparing for contract-salary negotiations. Which of the following job evaluation activities will give her the most useful bargaining data?

a. time studies
b. job analysis
c. factor valuation
d. compensable factors

Matching: Match the term to the activity which demonstrates the application of the term by placing the correlating letter in the space provided.

Activity

___ 8.17. Administration identified a nursing benchmark job to serve as a standard for other nursing positions.

___ 8.18. The committee is reviewing jobs to determine if jobs of similar demand receive equal pay.

___ 8.19. The consultant is observing employees at work and recording duties, responsibilities and the conditions under which the work is done.

___ 8.20. The salary and wage committee assigned codes to jobs of similar levels.

___ 8.21. The staff nurse and first level manager agree upon the personal requirements and capacities needed in the staff nurse's work.

___ 8.22. Nursing staff submit to administration a design for positions with clinical promotions.

Term

a. benchmark job

b. career ladders

c. point system

d. job analysis

e. job grades

f. job specifications

ANSWERS	TEXT REFERENCE
8.01. T	p. 158
8.02. F	p. 161
8.03. T	p. 165
8.04. d	p. 156
8.05. d	p. 149
8.06. a	p. 156, 157
8.07. a	p. 153
8.08. a	p. 161
8.09. b	p. 152
8.10. d	p. 152
8.11. c	p. 152
8.12. a	p. 152
8.13. f	p. 152
8.14. e	p. 154
8.15. b	p. 153, 156-159
8.16. c	p. 163
8.17. a	p. 152, 162
8.18. c	p. 164
8.19. d	p. 153, 154
8.20. e	p. 162
8.21. f	p. 152, 160
8.22. b	p. 150, 151

CHAPTER

9

Group Work and Team Building

The job of the nursing manager is to get work done through others. Therefore, every nurse manager must use groups to their maximum potential. The insights into group process given in this chapter will aid the nurse manager in facilitating positive group outcomes.

KEY TERMS

advisory committee
executive committee
group syntality
groupthink
linking pin
network
standing committee
weak links
working committee

OUTLINE

I. Introduction
   A. Group defined
   B. Group objectives
   C. Group functions

II. Linking pin structure
   A. Purpose
   B. Examples given

III. Standing committees
   A. Types
      1. Executive
      2. Working
      3. Advisory
   B. Place in organization
   C. Ad hoc committees
      1. Purpose
      2. Four advantages
      3. Three disadvantages

IV. Group communication
   A. Need for
   B. Contrasted with one-to-one communication
   C. Steps of communication process
   D. Size of the group
   E. Group syntality or cohesiveness
      1. Cohesive group characteristics
      2. Impact of group cohesiveness
   F. Reasons for joining the group

1. Admire group
2. Achieve desired end
3. Obtain protection

G. Groupthink
1. Defined
2. Negative effects
3. Symptoms
4. Minimizing techniques

F. Roles of group members
1. Leader
2. Idea generator
3. Evaluator
4. Problem solver
5. Moral supporter

G. Role of the leader
1. Prerequisites for leadership
2. Characteristics of leader
a. Investiture
b. Leadership style
(1). Autocratic
(2). Democratic
(3). Laissez faire
(4). relational:task orientation
3. Preparation for group leadership

H. Stages of group development
1. Forming
2. Storming
3. Norming
4. Performing
5. Adjourning

I. Communication network
1. Definitions
2. Formal and informal lines
3. Group shape impact
a. Circle
b. Chain
c. Fan
d. All channel

J. Summary of group communication

V. Analysis of group interaction
A. Categories for interaction analysis
B. Examples

VI. Managerial applications of group dynamics theory
A. Designing groups
B. Chairing groups
C. Serving as a group member

VII. Professional networking
A. Defined
B. Types
C. Requirement

VIII. Summary

CLASSROOM ACTIVITIES: Group Shapes and Communication

In the activities below chapter objective 4 will be role played. "Diagram the communication flow during a committee meeting to determine whether message transmission follows a fan, chain, circle, or all-channel pattern."

Time: 10 minutes for each group, followed by class discussion.

Choose 5 students per group.

Identify several short topics and assign one topic per group.
Possible topics:
Discuss the advantages and disadvantages of practicing a task oriented leadership style.
State three ways to reward a competent staff nurse.
State three ways to reduce sick leave use.

Arrange group chairs in the front of the classroom.

Instruct:
Group 1 to communicate as a circle group.
Group 2 to communicate as a chain group.
Group 3 to communicate as a Y group.

While each group explores the topic, the remainder of the class is to:
- diagram group communications,
- critique efficiency/effectiveness of group in relation to group design.

Discuss classroom observations.

CLASSROOM ACTIVITIES: Group Techniques

If students do not have a course in group process, the following two activities will give them opportunity to practice two group work techniques for future use.

NOMINAL GROUP TECHNIQUE

Time: 45 minutes

Introduction: The nominal group technique is a process which ensures the input of all group members, whether assertive or shy.

Identify topic: Possible topics: How can nursing attract capable students into nursing education? What can a health agency do to become a "preferred employer" and thus attract competent nurses?

Process

Each student is instructed to list his/her own ideas on a piece of paper.

Each group leader calls upon each group member to read one of his/her ideas.

The group leader records the idea on a blackboard or flip chart for all the group members to see. No judgment is made or shown by the group leader. The idea is simply recorded.

When all ideas have been elicited from *each* group member, the leader will repeat the cycle of calling upon group members to state ideas which have not yet been stated.

When ideas have been recorded, the group is asked to review the items. At this time clarification and some combining of items will occur.

The group will then be asked to vote for a given number of items by prioritizing them in writing.

The individual written prioritized items are then tabulated to determine the group priorities.

Technique strengths

Each group voice is heard, and group members equally contribute to the decision making process.

ASSIGNMENT: Group Process Analysis

Chapter objectives 3 and 4 may be used as an assignment for all levels of students.

Objective 3: Analyze the functions of a continuing group of which you are a member to identify the person who usually plays each of the following roles: leader, idea generator, evaluator, problem solver, and moral supporter.

Objective 4: Diagram the communication flow during a committee meeting to determine whether message transmission follows a fan, chain, circle, or all-channel pattern.

Activities

Identify a group of which you are a member.

State the purpose of the group and the number of group members.

Identify the group members who play each of the following roles: leader, idea generator, evaluator, problem solver, moral supporter.

For two of the above persons identify and describe the behaviors that support their roles.

Diagram the communication flow of the group. What type of communication pattern does the group follow?

How does the seating arrangement effect the communication flow?

ASSIGNMENT: Problems and Ad Hoc Committee

RN to BSN and graduate students who are familiar with an agency will profit from this assignment.

Objective 2: "Identify two problems in your organization for which an ad hoc committee is needed to investigate causes of those problems and suggest possible solutions.

Assignment

1. In one paragraph, as stated in objective, identify two problems which an ad hoc committee could appropriately address.
2. In one paragraph state reasons for preferring resolution by ad hoc committee(s).

TEST QUESTIONS

KNOWLEDGE AND COMPREHENSION

True : False

T F 9.01. Communication within a group is influenced by a member's motivation for joining.

T F 9.02. The major goals of a group are group consensus and group cohesiveness.

T F 9.03. A group in which minority opinions are regularly and freely expressed is usually more proficient in problem solving.

T F 9.04. Research indicates that communication network characteristics influence employee productivity and satisfaction.

Multiple Choice

9.05. The group member who characteristically asks for opinions, asks questions, mediates disagreements and gives interpretation is fulfilling what role in the group?
a. Leader.
b. Problem solver.
c. Idea generator.
d. Evaluator.

9.06. The nurse administrator who characteristically gives guiding suggestions and information to stimulate group members toward self-direction is practicing which of the following leadership styles:
a. autocratic.
b. democratic.
c. laissez faire.

9.07. Regardless of group shape (circle, fan, chain), the group leader is most likely to be the person:
a. at the "top" of the group structure.
b. who is the highest administrator/manager in the group.
c. placed in the most central position.
d. who is most peripheral in the group.

9.08. Principles of group communication derive from group characteristics including:
a. size.
b. composition.
c. structure.
d. all of above.

9.09. Nurse administrator Do Forme often appoints ad hoc committees to respond to specific problems. A potential advantage of this practice is that:
a. it supports the formal organizational structure.
b. ensures follow up of decisions thus promoting change.
c. ad hoc committees have executive power.
d. ad hoc committees utilize resources temporarily.

9.10. Which type group is likely to develop when assigned a complex task?
a. circle
b. chain
c. fan
d. all-channel

9.11. To effectively guide employees, a nurse manager must:
a. possess group skills
b. have in-depth knowledge of the matter at hand
c. practice consistency of leadership style
d. all of above

9.12. Speech, gestures, facial expressions, pictures and diagrams are all examples of which step of the communication process?
a. idea generation
b. message transmission
c. message receipt
d. feedback

9.13. Which of the following is/are most likely characteristic of a group of six members?
a. difficulty in reaching consensus
b. more productive than large groups
c. leaders influence group decisions
d. all of above

APPLICATION, ANALYSIS, AND/OR SYNTHESIS

Multiple Choice

9.14. Which of the following problems would best be handled by an ad hoc committee rather than by a standing committee?
a. selection of a new birthing bed.
b. audit of medication errors.
c. ongoing updating of infection control manual.
d. monitoring of implementation of the staffing pattern.

9.15. The quality circle recommends changes in the admissions process for outpatients. The quality circle is acting as a/an:
a. Ad hoc committee.
b. Advisory committee.
c. Executive committee.
d. Working committee.

9.16. The safety committee reviews all incident reports utilizing an audit form. The safety committee is acting as a/an:
a. Ad hoc committee.
b. Advisory committee.
c. Executive committee.
d. Working committee.

9.17. Nursing administration appointed a group to review patient care driven computer software. This group is acting as a/an:
a. Ad hoc committee.
b. Advisory committee.
c. Executive committee.
d. Working committee.

9.18. Nurse Unoit is supporting the ideas presented by Nurse Naivete. Nurse Wrkmore brings a written proposal to the committee meeting. Which group developmental stage is illustrated in the committee members behaviors?
a. forming
b. storming
c. norming
d. performing

9.19. Nurse Neutotown has recently accepted an administrative position in a distant city. She desires to develop helpful contacts through networking. Which of the following types of networks will be of benefit?
a. business
b. social and support
c. professional
d. all of above

9.20. Nurse executive observes that the committee in recent months seems to reflect the opinions of just two or three in the group. What can the nurse executive do to promote better individual input and quality of decisions?
a. compliment group on their cohesiveness
b. quickly implement the committee's recommendations
c. at each meeting, assign two members to "devil's advocate" role
d. all of above

Matching: Match the key terms to the appropriate illustrations by placing the letter in the space provided.

Illustrations

___ 9.21. The recently widowed nurse manager who finds support in in ad hoc committee is demonstrating which principle?

___ 9.22. Nurse manager of outpatient services is appointed to several committees.

___ 9.23. Nursing departments' organizational chart provides this.

___ 9.24. The entire committee rarely differs in opinions.

___ 9.25. The Tuesday group is charged with revising admission procedures this month.

___ 9.26. The administrator asked the Wednesday group to recommend a focus for community service.

___ 9.27. The public relations committee will be holding their regular meeting as scheduled.

Key Terms

a. advisory committee
b. communication network
c. group syntality
d. groupthink
e. linking pin
f. standing committee
g. weak link
h. working committee

ANSWERS	TEXT REFERENCE
9.01. T	p. 174
9.02. F	p. 169
9.03. T	p. 176
9.04. T	p. 177
9.05. b	p. 174
9.06. b	p. 175
9.07. c	p. 177, 178
9.08. d	p. 171
9.09. d	p. 170, 171
9.10. d	p. 177, 178
9.11. a	p. 17
9.12. b	p. 172
9.13. c	p. 172
9.14. a	p. 170, 171
9.15. b	p. 170
9.16. d	p. 170
9.17. a and/or b	p. 170, 171
9.18. d	p. 176
9.19. d	p. 179, 180
9.20. c	p. 173
9.21. g	p. 173
9.22. e	p. 170
9.23. b	p. 177
9.24. d	p. 173
9.25. h	p. 170
9.26. a	p. 170
9.27. f	p. 170

CHAPTER

10

Communication

Useful communication principles from various theorists and theories are presented in this chapter. Students will enjoy the application of transactional theory in the short classroom activities.

KEY TERMS

chain of command
double bind
frame of reference
homophyly
PAC diagrams
self preservation
transactional analysis

OUTLINE

I. Communication theorists and theories
 A. Berlo's linear model
  1. Source
  2. Message
  3. Channel
  4. Receiver
 B. Shannon and Weaver's circular model
  1. Signal
  2. Noise
  3. Feedback
 C. Fritz's emphasis upon communication climate
  1. Trust
  2. Message ambiguity
  3. Sender:receiver "prizing" one another
  4. Emotional separation
  5. Empathy between sender and receiver
  6. Perceived threat
  7. Fixed views
 D. Dance's helical model
  1. Impact of earlier messages
 E. Communication principles
  1. Communication is a two-way process
  2. Communication process can be impaired by "noise"
  3. Communication is both intrapersonal and interpersonal
  4. Communication is both verbal and nonverbal

- F. Social-psychological factors
  - 1. Homophyly
  - 2. Chain of command
  - 3. Frame of reference
  - 4. Self preservation
  - 5. Crisis
- G. Tuckman's stages of communication
  - 1. Forming
  - 2. Storming
  - 3. Norming
  - 4. Performing
- H. Research of communication consequences

II. Communication principles
- A. Seven principles
- B. Examples of principle application

III. Theory of transactional analysis
- A. Introduction
- B. Interpersonal transactions
  - 1. Interact to obtain positive or negative strokes
  - 2. Interact to maintain self-image
  - 3. Interaction as social functioning
- C. Types of interpersonal transactions
  - 1. Withdrawal
  - 2. Rituals
  - 3. Activities
  - 4. Pastimes
  - 5. Games
  - 6. Intimacy
- D. Structural analysis
  - 1. Parent
  - 2. Adult
  - 3. Child
- E. Laws governing interpersonal transactions
  - 1. Described
  - 2. Types
    - a. Complementary
    - b. Crossed
    - c. Duplex
  - 3. PAC diagrams
- F. Harris:Life positions
  - 1. I'm not OK; you're OK
  - 2. I'm not OK; you're not OK
  - 3. I'm OK; you're not OK
  - 4. I'm OK; you're OK

IV. Management applications for transactional analysis
- A. Effective patterns
  - 1. Complementary
  - 2. Adult-Adult
  - 3. Nurturing Parent-Child
- B. Ineffective patterns
  - 1. Not OK
    - a. Child
    - b. Parent
  - 2. Predisposition through nursing education practices
    - a. Overdeveloped Adult
    - b. Alcoholic game
    - c. Exaggerated Parent
    - d. Neglected Child
  - 3. Physician:Parent-Nurse:Child
  - 4. Nurse-patient's changing state
- C. Usefulness
  - 1. Modify behavior to increase productivity
  - 2. Increase worker's problem-solving ability
  - 3. Interpret and modify self responses

V. Communication levels
- A. Top level uses "Broadcast" system
- B. Second level uses formal information systems
- C. Third level uses supplementary and interpersonal communications
- D. Fourth level instrumental systems
- E. Strengthen communication using informational:relational aspects
  - 1. Improving informational aspects
  - 2. Improving relational aspects
- F. Guidelines to improve communication

VI. Organizational double bind
- A. Double bind examples
- B. Sources
- C. Minimizing double bind

VII. Documentation of care
- A. Importance of
- B. Weakness of
- C. Inhibiting factors
- D. Facilitating factors

VIII. Management information systems
- A. Use
- B. Impact

IX. Summary

CLASSROOM ACTIVITY: Communication Analysis Using Transaction Analysis Theory

This activity will meet chapter objective 2: "While observing two employees during a heated interchange, diagram several of their interpersonal communications to reveal which verbal transactions were parallel and which were crossed."

ACTIVITY I

Time: 5 minutes for staged argument
10 minutes for classroom discussion

Identify a topic about which classroom members have strongly differing opinions; e.g., the hospital should have a policy requiring O.R. nurses to participate in abortions; nursing homes should house patients with AIDS in double rooms with patients who do not have AIDS.

Choose two vocal students, one pro and one con regarding the topic.

Privately instruct the two students that they are to express their views and include a heated exchange in front of the class for a period of about five minutes. If the second part is also used, tell the students that you will interrupt them at the end of their time.

Introduce the activity to the class: "I've asked *student* and *student* to share their ideas regarding *topic*. As they are sharing their positions, note the types of exchanges that occur. Diagram these exchanges using transactional analysis theory and PAC diagrams."

During discussion, draw from the class examples of crossed and parallel communications. Ask class members to identify the results of the crossed and parallel communications.

ACTIVITY II

Addition of the following will incorporate the first chapter objective as well.

Time: 5 minutes

As the above discussion/argument between the students is heated and time is nearing an end, interrupt the exchange by simply saying "stop" and "stay as you are" or "freeze—do not move." At this point ask students to identify parent, adult and/or child nonverbal behaviors. Ask students to note defensive nonverbal behaviors on the part of presenting students and class observers as well.

Thank the presenters and tell the class that they were instructed to get into a heated exchange and proceed to the diagramming of communications.

Diagram 3-5 of the student exchanges.
What patterns became predominant?
What type of communication was occurring when the exchange became heated?

ASSIGNMENT: Analysis of personal communication

Objective 1 is carried out in the assignment. "Diagram the direction of your verbal and nonverbal interpersonal messages to others during the course of a committee meeting."

ACTIVITY

1. Write a journal of five interactions with a specific individual. Use the following format.

Time	Communicator	Time	Communication	Noise

2. Analyze communication; e.g.,
   a. What messages were heard?
   b. What interfered with communications?
   c. What were the results when communications were properly heard?
   d. What were the results when communications were not correctly heard?

TEST QUESTIONS

KNOWLEDGE AND COMPREHENSION

True : False

T F 10.01. Harris claims that once a child has selected a life position, s/he operates from that position throughout life.

T F 10.02. An advantage of computer information systems is the large quantity of information available to all nurse managers.

Multiple Choice

10.03. Berlo's linear model of communication identified four elements for each communicating act. They are:
a. source, message, channel, receiver.
b. sender, mode, nonverbal message, destination.
c. trust, sender, receiver, mode.
d. noise, trust, source, receiver.

10.04. The purpose of feedback is:
a. promotion of trust.
b. refining the message.
c. to show "prizing" of another.
d. to demonstrate empathy.

10.05. According to Klatt, when administration distributes a bulletin to all employees administration is using:
a. top level broadcast system.
b. formal information systems.
c. supplementary communication systems.
d. instrumental communications.

10.06. In the alcoholic game, which of the following behaviors characterize the rescuer?
a. attributes behavior of alcoholic to physiological defect
b. provides the alcoholic beverage
c. alienates family and friends
d. behaves unwisely

Matching: Match the theorists or theory to the contribution by placing the appropriate letter in the space provided.

		Contribution	Theorists/Theory
____	10.07.	emphasis on communication climate	a. Berlo
____	10.08.	linear model of communication	b. Dance
____	10.09.	circular model of communication	c. Drucker
____	10.10.	helical model of communication	d. Fritz
____	10.11.	identified stages of communication	e. Shannon and Weaver
____	10.12.	emphasis is on receiver	f. transactional
____	10.13.	parent, child, adult aspects of personality	g. Tuckman

APPLICATION, ANALYSIS, AND/OR SYNTHESIS

Multiple Choice

In questions 10.14 - 10.17 principles from communication theories are being practiced. Identify the theory to which the practiced principle(s) relate(s).

10.14. Nurse I. Tolyu sent a memo instructing staff.
   a. Berlo's linear model of communication
   b. transactional analysis child aspect of personality
   c. Tuckman's stages of communication
   d. principles identified by Fritz

10.15. Nurse manager R. E. Flect in talking with a staff nurse said, "What I hear you saying is . . . . "
   a. Dance
   b. Shannon and Weaver
   c. Berlo
   d. Tuckman

10.16. New nurse manager Wiseman will wait to present the proposal to administration until after a trusting working relationship is established with administration.
   a. transactional analysis parent-child communications
   b. Drucker
   c. Fritz
   d. Shannon and Weaver

10.17. The staff nurses sighed with relief and expressed a willingness to proceed.
   a. Berlo
   b. Shannon and Weaver
   c. Fritz
   d. Tuckman

10.18. The nurse manager stands with hands on hips, frowns, and shakes her head from side to side. These nonverbal behaviors indicate that the nurse manager is practicing which state according to transactional analysis theory?
a. parent
b. adult
c. child

10.19. On the employee evaluation forms the nurse is described as being intuitive, creative, and spontaneous. According to transactional analysis theory, which state is the employee most likely practicing?
a. parent
b. adult
c. child

10.20. Two staff nurses can no longer communicate. Which is the most likely communication pattern they have practiced?
a. child:child
b. adult:child, child:adult
c. parent:child, adult:parent

10.21. Two staff nurses demonstrate longstanding good communication. To achieve this which of the following communication patterns have they most likely practiced?
a. parent:parent
b. adult:adult
c. child:child
d. all of above

10.22. The physician instructs a competent nurse in an elementary manner. This is an example of which of the following communication patterns?
a. physician: parent:parent, nurse: parent:parent
b. physician: adult:child, nurse: adult:child
c. physician: adult:adult, nurse: child:child
d. physician: parent:child, nurse: adult:adult

10.23. The patient is improving and wants to be included in the decision making about her own care. The nurse, however, continues to tell the patient what to do. What communication pattern is occurring?
a. nurse: parent:child, patient: adult:adult
b. nurse: adult:adult, patient: adult:adult
c. nurse: child:parent, patient: parent:child
d. nurse: adult:parent, patient: parent:adult

10.24. The young nurse needs support from an older nurse manager who feels threatened by the young nurses proposals for change. The young nurse is experiencing:
a. self preservation
b. homophyly
c. double bind
d. all of above

10.25. The nurse manager wants to increase completeness and accuracy of nurse documentation. Which of the following will likely aid better documentation?
a. vital sign flow charts at bedside
b. a designated room for all charting activities
c. use of incidence reports when documentation is complete
d. all of above

ANSWERS	TEXT REFERENCE
10.01. T	p. 192
10.02. F	p. 197
10.03. a	p. 182
10.04. b	p. 183
10.05. a	p. 194
10.06. a	p. 192
10.07. d	p. 182
10.08. a	p. 183
10.09. e	p. 183
10.10. b	p. 183
10.11. g	p. 183
10.12. c	p. 189
10.13. f	p. 186
10.14. a	p. 182
10.15. b	p. 183
10.16. c	p. 183
10.17. d	p. 186
10.18. a	p. 190
10.19. c	p. 190
10.20. c	p. 191, 193
10.21. d	p. 191
10.22. d	p. 191, 193
10.23. a	p. 191, 193
10.24. c	p. 195, 296
10.25. a	p. 196

CHAPTER

11

Time Management

Time use analysis incorporates each of the steps of the management process. Time logs (see Figure 11.1 at the end of this *Manual*) assist in *gathering data* of how time is used. Analysis of the gathered data, as it relates to position and/or unit goals, objectives, and categories, leads to *problem identification* regarding time use. Comparison of activity time needs in relation to available time resources becomes an important *planning* tool. Time parameters for productivity communicate certain expectancies thus providing *direction* to staff. Finally, time analysis can be an *evaluative* process used to *prevent* nonproductive time use.

KEY TERMS

activity wheel
critical path
delegation
Gantt chart
PERT diagram
procrastination

OUTLINE

- I. Introduction
  - A. Manager's time
  - B. Controlling time
    1. Clarify work goals
    2. Set priorities
    3. Identify activities for goal achievement
    4. Secure resources
    5. Schedules time and follows schedule
- II. Analyzing present time use
  - A. Keep time log in half-hour intervals
  - B. Categorize recorded activities
  - C. Analyze findings
  - D. Personality characteristic influences
    1. Goal centered
    2. Plan oriented
    3. Completion focused
    4. Emphasis centered
    5. Limits sensitive
- III. Setting and prioritizing goals
  - A. Goal perspectives
    1. High, moderate, or trivial priority
    2. Daily prioritizing
    3. Long term, intermediate, short term
  - B. Devise written plan and schedule

1. Regular time blocking
2. Matrix decision making

IV. Gantt Chart
   A. Defined
   B. Example
      1. Activities identified
      2. Time schedule plotted

V. Performance evaluation and review technique (PERT)
   A. Addition of three time estimates
      1. Pessimistic
      2. Probable
      3. Optimistic
   B. PERT Diagram example
      1. Optimistic path
      2. Probable path
      3. Critical path
   C. PERT Activity Chart

VI. Delegation
   A. Defined
   B. Reasons for failing to delegate
      1. "Soft" operating information
      2. Unwillingness/inability to share information
      3. Lack of confidence in subordinates
      4. Fear of loosing control
      5. Reluctance - may appear incompetent
   B. What should and should **NOT** be delegated
      1. Do **NOT** delegate strategic planning
      2. Do **NOT** delegate evaluation or discipline immediate subordinates
      3. Do delegate responsibility for total project
   C. Delegation as a legal contract
      1. Manager and delegatee agreement
      2. Written contract

VII. Time traps
   A. Activity wheel
      1. Defined
      2. Prescriptive behaviors
         a. Set behavioral goals
         b. Construct a Gantt or PERT chart
         c. Monitor programs
   B. Procrastination
      1. Defined
      2. Arising out of fear of failure
   C. Interruptions
      1. "Open door" policy
         a. Control drop-in visits
         b. Schedule regular information meetings
         c. Send weekly updated information to superiors
      2. Telephone calls
         a. Eliminate social conversation
         b. Prepare agenda for phone calls
         c. Train secretary to screen calls
         d. Provide routine operating information
         e. Schedule formal appointments
   D. Committee work
      1. Apply group process theory
      2. Schedule meetings to facilitate attendance
      3. Advance dissemination of written agenda
      4. Timely circulation of meeting minutes

VIII. Saying no
   A. Impact of
      1. "To do" nursing orientation
      2. Crisis nursing orientation
      3. Failure to plan
   B. Four reasons to say "no"
   C. When to say no

IX. Schedules
   A. Calendar
   B. Daily to-do lists
   C. Tickler file
   D. Scheduled "R and R" days
   E. Work perspective

X. Summary

ASSIGNMENT: Time Log Analysis

This assignment fulfills the first chapter objective and integrates chapter objectives 1, 2, and 3.

Objective 1: Keep a daily time log for one week and tally time spent in each task component of your job.

Objective 2: Write three long-term and three short-term personal goals and rank these in order of priority.

Objective 3: Identify two activities that will promote the achievement of your highest priority long-range goal and two activities that will promote the achievement of your highest priority short-range goal.

Figure 11.1 (at the end of this *Manual*) may be copied and distributed to students for keeping a time log. Principles of assessing time use that are discussed in the text are incorporated in the log; log in half-hour intervals, identify the category of each activity, identify the priority level of the activities, and relate time use to goals. Analysis of the activities is facilitated through the category, priority, and goal columns and the suggested coding at the bottom of the log. Note that the category column may be used to address either the management process for students who are nurse managers or the nursing process for students who are not in management positions.

Activities

1. State one long range, one medium-range, and one short-term goal which relates to your position.
2. Keep a time log using Figure 11.1 for _?_ days.
3. Assign appropriate category, priority, and goal codes to each activity.
4. Subtotal daily time consumed by activities for each *CATEGORY*.
5. Subtotal daily time consumed by activities in each *PRIORITY* level.
6. Subtotal daily time spent in activities supporting the identified long range, medium-range, and short-term goals.

Analysis

1. Critique the distribution of category time use.

   Does each category occur?

   If not, should the absent categories be included?

   How could you better distribute time use among the categories?

2. Note priority levels.

   How much of your time was used in "L" or "X" priority activities?

   Are there any identifiable repeating patterns of activities that could be eliminated?

   How could you reduce "L" and "X" activities?

   (Nurse managers:

   What is the employer's cost per minute for your time?

   What is the average daily cost of "L" and "X" activities?)

3. Examine the activities which support the identified goals.

   Do activities appropriately support EACH of the goals?

   Is the time proportionately spent among the goals?

   What would you like to do differently to better support the goals?

ADDITIONAL WRITTEN ASSIGNMENTS

1. Chapter Objective 4: Plan your personal time schedule so as to provide a four hour time block each week for activities that support your high-priority goals.

   Generic BSN students will find the assignment useful.

2. Chapter Objective 5: Develop a Gantt chart to guide a group of nurses through a complex, multistage project.

   The development of a Gantt chart will require higher level skills and thus is an assignment which is more appropriate for graduate level students.

3. Chapter Objective 6: Analyze your work habits to identify two common time traps and develop a plan to insulate yourself against both.

This objective is useful for all levels of students—and faculty, too.

ROLE PLAY: Just Say "No"

Time: 10 minutes plus discussion

Preparation: Two copies of the script.
Read the **background situation** to the class.
Ask for a volunteer Nurse Manager, and a volunteer Nurse Imhelpful.
Give script copies to volunteers.

Situation:

Background: Patient documentation has been a long-term problem. The nurse administrator, at last, has stimulated the interest of the administrator in portable computer terminals for use in patient documentation. The administrator has asked the nurse administrator to submit an outline proposal stating what is desired, why, and cost:benefit analysis in 48 hours.

(Role play)

Current: (Nurse administrator is working on the proposal at her desk behind closed door.)

Nurse Imhelpful: (Pops into the nurse administrator's office and starts talking enthusiastically.) "Hi, you know that PCA procedure which has been such a problem? Well, several of us were talking about it and we came up with some good ideas. Just wait until you hear them.....

Responses:

Option 1:

Nurse Administrator: (Looking up from paper strewn desk with pencil in hand INTERRUPTS) "I'm very busy right now, Please come back later."

Nurse Imhelpful: (Respond the way you feel both verbally and nonverbally.)

Option 2:

Nurse Imhelpful: (Repeat bursting into office as above.)

Nurse Administrator: (Look up. Remain seated.) "Hmmm, that sounds interesting, but right now I'm busy with a proposal...

Nurse Imhelpful: (INTERRUPTS) "Oh, this won't take but a few minutes."

Nurse Manager: (Sighs) "I can't now."

Nurse Imhelpful: (Respond as you feel and leave office.)

Option 3:

Nurse Imhelpful: (Repeat bursting into office as above.)

Nurse Manager: (Stand up and move away from desk to acknowledge Nurse Imhelpful. Look directly at Nurse Imhelpful.) "Hmmm, that's great. Let's schedule a time when the group can go over the ideas you have. Could you write down the ideas and slip them under my door the day before we get together so I can have a chance to think them over?

(Walks over to wall calendar and without pausing says:) How about meeting on Friday or Monday?

Time is scheduled.

(Nurse Manager walks Nurse Imhelpful to door.)

Nurse Imhelpful: (Respond verbally and nonverbally as you feel.)

Discussion:

1. What was heard in each scenario?
2. What did nonverbal behaviors convey?
3. Contrast and critique the Nurse Manager's responses.

   What did she do that caused problems?

   What did she do right?

   How did Nurse Imhelpful feel in each situation?

TEST QUESTIONS

KNOWLEDGE AND COMPREHENSION

True : False

T F 11.01. The higher a manager's position, the more time is controlled by others.

T F 11.02. A manager who delegates easily will find that additional time is consumed by the need to supervise the delegated activity.

T F 11.03 Research has shown that using contracts for delegated activities is unnecessary.

Multiple Choice

11.04. Effective planning and scheduling of the nurse manager's time *begins* with:
a. responding to mail and memos
b. participative management
c. establishing priorities
d. designing a staff scheduling model to meet institutional needs

11.05. When prioritizing goals the nurse manager will
a. identify long, intermediate, and short range goals
b. rank goals as high, moderate, and low priority
c. prioritize goals on a daily basis
d. all of above

11.06. PERT differs from other planning techniques in:
a. using time estimates for each activity
b. combing several planning steps to facilitate time use
c. focusing on who is accountable for each identified activity
d. all of above

11.07. An "open door" management philosophy means that you as manager:
a. invite staff to come to your office any time
b. include staff in all decision making
c. make time available to staff to discuss needs
d. see staff by appointments only

11.08. A major key to controlling interruptions is:
a. identifying and addressing reoccurring interruptions
b. practicing a schedule open door policy
c. seeing people by appointment
d. all of above

11.09. This tool is especially useful in evaluating progress of several activities that are carried out simultaneously to eventually come together to meet a goal at a target date.
a. Time log
b. Gantt chart
c. PERT diagram
d. Activity log

APPLICATION, ANALYSIS, AND/OR SYNTHESIS

Multiple Choice

11.10. Nurse Ildoit is determined to achieve a high priority intermediate level goal. Which of the following behaviors will support *responsible* goal achievement?

a. Nurse Ildoit asks her secretary to block out Tuesday morning on the appointment calendar.
b. Nurse Ildoit closes the office door and tells the secretary to see that she is not interrupted.
c. Nurse Ildoit focuses the major portion of her time on the goal.
d. all of above

11.11. Which of the following are necessary activities when using a Gantt Chart to guide development of a new eye outpatient surgery service?

a. Write relevant nursing policies and procedures.
b. Calculate numbers and categories of staff.
c. Conduct market survey to determine potential need and use of services.
d. all of above

11.12. Delegation is a major management tool. Which is a positive guide to appropriate delegation?

a. Delegate task responsibility, but maintain authority to ensure a quality outcome.
b. Delegate task responsibility and authority, but closely monitor task progress.
c. Both task responsibility and authority must be delegated at equivalent levels.
d. None of the above.

11.13. Useful analysis of a time log will include which of the following?

1. activities listed in 15 minute intervals
2. relationship of activities to goals
3. categorization of activities
4. priority level of activities

a. 1, 2
b. 2, 3
c. 2, 3, 4
d. all of above

11.14. To use time well, you will want to do each of the following. In what order will you do them?

1. delegate activities
2. identify goals to be achieved
3. identify activities that can and cannot be concurrently achieved
4. identify time lines for activities
5. identify activities needed to achieve goals

a. 1, 2, 3, 4, 5
b. 1, 2, 5, 3, 4
c. 2, 3, 4, 5, 1
d. 2, 5, 3, 4, 1

11.15. Which of the following telephone conversations should be eliminated in the interest of time utilization?

a. "I'm calling to ask if you have any questions or addition regarding the ad hoc committee agenda."
b. "How did your son's birthday surprise go last night? Did the other kids like it too?"
c. "I would like to meet with you this week to go over your proposal. I need to better understand the second section."
d. "I have received a complaint about the care Nurse X gave patient Z. Will you please check into the situation? Can you meet with me about this Tuesday at 2:00 p.m.

11.16. The head nurses are grumbling about the time wasted in committee meetings. The nurse administrator wants to encourage participative management. Which of the following are recommended activities for the nurse administrator in this situation?

a. require that she give permission before a meeting can be held
b. analyze group dynamics
c. eliminate non-productive committees
d. chair the committees

11.17. The staff nurse asks the nurse manager to alter the schedule in a way which is against the contract. The nurse manager's best response is:
  a. "Let's talk about that later."
  b. "Come to my office and we'll look over the schedule."
  c. "No, I can not do that."
  d. none of the above

11.18. Nursing managers receive little reinforcement from "outside". A helpful time management tool which can also serve as a reinforcement tool is:
  a. a scheduling calendar
  b. prioritizing tomorrow's tasks
  c. defensive administration practices
  d. a "to-do" list that records accomplishments

ANSWERS	TEXT REFERENCE
11.01. T	p. 200
11.02. F	p. 205
11.03. F	p. 206
11.04. c	p. 201, 202
11.05. d	p. 202
11.06. a	p. 203
11.07. c	p. 207
11.08. d	p. 207
11.09. b	p. 202
11.10. a	p. 202
11.11. d	p. 203
11.12. c	p. 205
11.13. c	p. 201
11.14. d	p. 201, 202, 203
11.15. b	p. 207
11.16. b	p. 207
11.17. c	p. 208
11.18. d	p. 208

CHAPTER

12

Staffing

The task of staffing incorporates each of the steps identified in systems theory and the management process. In addition, staffing requires the synthesis of agency mission, philosophy, objectives and knowledge of trends, societal, nursing, and health care. Staffing a unit of Podville Hospital is presented as an ongoing group classroom project in chapters 12 through 20 producing an end product of a staffing pattern. As the project evolves from class to class students have the opportunity to apply the theories and guidelines presented in the text in a very real way.

KEY TERMS

case management
critical path
direct care
functional
FTE
indirect care
interrater reliability
modular staffing
patient classification
primary care
team nursing

OUTLINE

I. Overview of staffing system
  A. Nine interdependent actions for staffing
  B. Advantages of uniform staffing
    1. Easier to administer
    2. Prevent excessive transfers
    3. Facilitate contract negotiations
  C. Identify staffing philosophy
  D. Identify staffing objectives

II. Methods of assigning personnel
  A. Functional
    1. Description
    2. Advantage
    3. Disadvantages
      a. Fragmented care
      b. Depersonalized care
  B. Team
    1. Description
    2. Composition
    3. Pitfalls
  C. Primary nursing
    1. Description

2. All RN staff rationale
3. Role of head nurse

D. Modular
1. Description
2. Forming pairs or trios
3. Assignment
4. Role of professional nurse

E. Nursing case management
1. Definition
2. Objectives
3. Case manager role
a. Responsibilities
b. Tools
(1). Case management plan
(2). Critical path diagram
c. Implementation examples

III. Predicting staffing needs
A. Methods
1. Nurse:patient ratios
2. Work-time analysis
3. Management engineering methods

B. Rationale for proper staffing
1. Cost containment
a. Reasons for nursing personnel cuts
(1). Largeness of nursing budget
(2). Nursing lacks voice and power
b. Ongoing staff:patient needs adjustments
2. Promote morale
3. Promote staffing stability

IV. Systems approach to staffing
A. Input
1. Patient classification
2. Staff capabilities
B. Throughput
C. Output
D. Controls
E. Feedback loops

V. Predicting nursing workload
A. Overview
B. Patient census
1. Variations
2. Average daily census
3. Patient services
4. Psychological workload
5. Average length of stay
6. Admissions reservations
7. Seasonal adjustments
8. Impact on staffing

B. Patient care needs
1. Direct care
2. Indirect care
3. Ministerial care
4. Health teaching
5. Example of determining needs
a. Identify potential types of patients
b. Identify needed nursing activities
c. Sample time required to per form activities
d. Set time standards

C. Direct care
1. Quantify direct nursing care
a. Self-report
b. Observation
2. Limitations to quantifying nursing care

D. Patient classification systems
1. Defined
2. Purpose
3. Four category example
4. Interrater reliability

E. Indirect care
1. Activities
2. Example
F. Health teaching
G. Work sampling

VI. Determining personnel levels and types
A. Rational for all RN staff
B. Consideration of certified specialists
C. Impact of outside agencies
1. Cost containment
2. JCAHO standards

VII. Determining the number of staff
A. Absent days
B. Calculations
C. Comparisons

VIII. Summary

CLASSROOM GROUP PROJECT: Staffing Podville Hospital's Pediatrics Unit

The activities for the staffing project incorporate chapter objectives 1 and 2.

Objective 1: Diagram the staffing system in your nursing organization to reveal three inputs, two throughput paths, three outputs, and two feedback loops for the system.

Objective 2: Identify two subsystems within the nurse staffing system for your nursing organization (perhaps use of supplementary agency personnel, registry employees, or travelling nurses), with input, throughput, and output elements for each.

Time: 45 minutes (Additional activities for subsequent chapters will build on the following activities.)

Situation: Podville Hospital is a large research and teaching hospital which draws from a large geographic region. An overview of the organizational structure of the nursing department is presented in Figure 7.2 (at the end of this *Manual*). The pediatrics unit includes several services and is illustrated in Figure 12.1 (at the end of this *Manual*). The use of an overhead of Figure 12.1 will facilitate sharing needed background information.

Note that the pediatric services include general medical-surgical, intensive care, infectious problems, and a 10-bed short-term stay unit. The short-term stay unit provides extended care for "outpatients" and "recovery" up to 12 hours. In addition the short-term unit provides respite care and overnight care for children of night shift nurses. Both respite care and overnight care use a reservation system.

Podville Hospital Administration is committed to facilitating quality care through the use of clinical specialists and a pediatric clinical specialist is housed on the unit. Podville Hospital has also adapted a patient care driven computer system. The unit clerk responsibilities include computer input and output for the unit.

Activities: Defining (additional) inputs needed for staffing pediatrics

1. What are the institutional philosophies and values that impact staffing decisions?
2. Consider:

   How the facility structure influences staffing model to be designed.

   How patient care needs are to be defined.

   What is the use pattern of each of the services?

   What type of staff are available?

   What might be built into the pattern to stabilize nursing staff?

3. Podville Hospital must function within given regulations.

   What JCAHO guidelines should be considered?

   Does the hospital insurance carrier specify conditions related to staffing?

   Identify (create) union contract specifications that pertain to staffing.

   What are the hospital-wide staffing policies? (Consider the benefits - holidays, sick days, vacation days, staff development days, etc.)

These inputs will be a foundation upon which the group will build to develop a staffing pattern for the Pediatric unit at Podville Hospital. When considering the management process, the inputs are part of the data collection that will guide needs identification and planning.

ASSIGNMENT: Staffing Problem and Solution

Chapter objectives 1 and 3 are incorporated in the assignment.

Objective 1: Diagram the staffing system in your nursing organization to reveal three inputs, two throughput paths, three outputs, and two feedback loops for the system.

Objective 3: Interview a nurse manager in your agency to determine her or his opinions about the advantages and disadvantages of the current method for nursing assignment (functional, team primary, modular, case).

(Generic BSN students could be assigned an interview while RN students could identify a staffing problem which effects his/her own unit.)

Activities

1. Identify a staffing problem either through interview or your own experience. Briefly describe the problem.
2. Diagram the staffing (sub)system of which the problem is a part. Identify the inputs, throughput paths, outputs, and feedback loops.
3. Describe the parts of the diagram that impact the problem.

   Does the problem exist because the staffing system structure is not followed or is selectively followed?

   Does the problem exist because of a lack in the staffing system structure?
4. What recommendations would you make to resolve the identified problem? Do consider solutions beyond that of hiring additional staff.

TEST QUESTIONS

KNOWLEDGE AND COMPREHENSION

True : False

T F 12.01. Staffing policies should be applied uniformly in all units.

T F 12.02. A case manager is responsible for giving direct care to her patient load.

T F 12.03. Nursing staff are demoralized when work load and staff are unbalanced.

T F 12.04. Research demonstrates that nurses' psychological workload decreases with shorter patient stays.

T F 12.05. Matching patient care needs with employees' abilities maximizes worker productivity and patient satisfaction.

T F 12.06. When calculating the number of RNs needed, the nurse manager needs to count 1.10 persons per position.

Multiple Choice

12.07. To minimize misunderstandings regarding staffing practices managers should:
- a. develop a staffing philosophy.
- b. consistently follow the same staffing pattern.
- c. encourage each unit to do its own staffing.
- d. all of above.

12.08. An advantage of functional assignment of personnel is:
- a. decrease in communication requirements between staff levels.
- b. staff become expert in assignment area.
- c. continuity of patient care.
- d. all of above.

12.09. To promote continuity of patient care using a staff which includes RNs, LPNs, and aides, which staffing model would be preferable?
- a. modular
- b. team
- c. primary
- d. functional
- e. case management

12.10. Which of the following are characteristics of a PRIMARY method of nurse staffing?
1. all RN staff
2. 24-hour responsibility for patient care
3. same nurse:patient assignment throughout patient stay
4. is less expensive than team or functional nursing

- a. 1, 2, 3
- b. 2, 3, 4
- c. 1, 2, 4
- d. all of above

Matching: Match the systems step with the appropriate staffing activity by placing the letter in the space provided.

Activity

____ 12.11. unit nursing personnel roster

____ 12.12. complexity of patient care needs

____ 12.13. labor contracts

____ 12.14. average daily patient census

____ 12.15. shift-by-shift patient census **forecast**

____ 12.16. computerized reports indicating number of sick days used per employee

____ 12.17. number of each personnel category needed

____ 12.18. orienting employee to job responsibilities

____ 12.19. staff member capabilities

____ 12.20. JCAHO standards

Systems Step

a. input

b. process

c. output

d. controls

e. feedback

APPLICATION, ANALYSIS, AND/OR SYNTHESIS

Multiple Choice

12.21. Advantages of a modular nurse staffing pattern include:
a. promotes continuity of care
b. utilizes all level of personnel appropriately
c. promotes "bonding" of RN and assistant
d. all of above

12.22. Staffing includes the total process of matching resources to needs. The following are each activities which need to be done to facilitate the best use of human resources. In what order will the nurse manager see that these are done?
1. determine categories and numbers of nursing personnel needed
2. design a staffing pattern by unit and shifts
3. determine method of personnel as signment
4. recruit and select personnel to fill available positions
5. identify type and amount of nursing care to be given
6. assign responsibilities

a. 1, 2, 3, 4, 5, 6
b. 2, 4, 3, 5, 1, 6
c. 3, 2, 1, 4, 5, 6
d. 4, 1, 3, 2, 5, 6

12.23. The nurse manager of the new outpatient eye services is to submit staffing recommendations. Which of the following will she need to consider?
a. type of patient care needed
b. type of staffing expertise needed for that care
c. cost-effective staffing; i.e., difference in reimbursement from on type patient to another
d. all of above

12.24. Which of the following approaches would produce the most accurate assessment of number and mix of staff needed?
a. a system based upon DRGs
b. a system based upon number of actual patient care days
c. a system based upon care units needed by the patient
d. a mixture of DRGs and patient care days

12.25. Which of the following is an example of *direct* care in contrast to indirect care?
a. Nurse Matilda participates in the infection control committee.
b. Nurse Mod Ern attends a meeting to review nursing care plans.
c. Nurse Beulah teaches patient how to change dressings.
d. Nurse Fus Budgette audits the patient incident reports for failure to practice safety rules.

Matching: Match the assignment method to the characteristic of the assignment method by placing the appropriate letter in the space provided.

		Assignment Characteristic	Assignment Method
____	12.26.	Nurse Doit and nursing assistant Metoo are assigned total patient care for eight patients on the medical unit.	a. case management b. functional c. modular d. primary e. team
____	12.27.	Unit 1 assigned two RNs to medication administration, 1 RN and 1 LPN to treatments and therapies, and nursing assistants to personal care.	
____	12.28.	Nurse Carefor is assigned total care for patients throughout their stay.	
____	12.29.	Nurse Helpinghand planned and coordinated care for Teddy from emergency room, pediatrics, surgery and discharge.	
____	12.30.	The new pediatric unit assigned one RN, two LPNs, and three nursing assistants to each wing.	

ANSWERS	TEXT REFERENCE
12.01. T	p. 214
12.02. F	p. 218
12.03. T	p. 220
12.04. F	p. 222, 223
12.05. T	p. 229
12.06. F	p. 224
12.07. a	p. 214
12.08. b	p. 215
12.09. a	p. 218
12.10. d	p. 217
12.11. c	p. 221
12.12. a	p. 221
12.13. d	p. 221
12.14. a	p. 221
12.15. b	p. 221
12.16. e	p. 221
12.17. c	p. 221
12.18. b	p. 221
12.19. a	p. 221
12.20. d	p. 221
12.21. d	p. 218
12.22. d	p. 229, 231
12.23. d	p. 224, 225, 231
12.24. c	p. 224
12.25. c	p. 224
12.26. c	p. 218
12.27. b	p. 215, 216
12.28. d	p. 217
12.29. a	p. 218
12.30. e	p. 216, 217

CHAPTER

13

Recruitment, Selection, Orientation

Recruiting, selecting and orienting nurses in an era of fast paced medical practices and constant technical and regulatory changes offers its own very special challenges. The understanding and use of the guidelines presented in this chapter will contribute in creating an effective recruitment, selection and orientation processes.

KEY TERMS

bounties
induction training
internship
product
marketing
orientation
placement
preceptor
product
promotion
recruitment
selection

OUTLINE

I. Introduction
   A. Definition of recruitment
   B. Staffing of nurse recruitment
   B. Characteristics of nurse recruiter
II. Constructing a nursing personnel profile
   A. Ten items to profile
   B. Critique of existing profile
III. Planning a recruitment program
   A. Exit interviews
      1. Conduct
      2. Review
      3. Problem identification
      4. Caution
   B. Marketing
      1. Defined
      2. Concepts
         a. Product
         b. Place
         c. Promotion
         d. Price
   C. Recruitment plan
      1. Annual review
      2. Data base

a. Workload
b. Organizational changes
3. Governmental data
4. Determine number and types of area graduating nurses
5. Compare offerings with competitors
a. Capitalize on differences
b. Promote correction of negative differences
6. Examine outcomes of previous recruitment activities

IV. Traditional recruitment methods
A. Advertising
1. Efficacy of local advertising
2. Matching journal to position
B. Career days
C. Recruitment literature
1. Content
2. Distribution
3. Types
D. Open house
1. Physical plant
2. Invitations
3. Activities
E. Continuing education programs
1. Rationale for use
2. Exposure to facility
3. Availability of information
4. Presence of nurse recruiter
F. Employee referrals
1. Employee recruits
2. Bounties

V. Ad Hoc recruitment methods
A. Present positives
B. Temporary staffing
1. Outside agency use
2. In-house staffing agency
3. Travelling nurses
C. "Headhunters"

VI. Processing and interviewing applicants
A. Timely processing
B. Selection of contact personnel
C. Interviewer responsibilities
D. Selecting interviewer
E. Interviewing
1. Preparation
2. Process
3. Principles
4. Environment
a. Physical
b. Comfort
c. Time
d. Interaction
5. Content

VII. Selection
A. Selection defined
B. Placement defined

VIII. Comparing backgrounds of job applicants
A. Need
B. Example
C. Methods
D. Weighing applicants' personal characteristics
1. Appearance
2. Manner of speech
3. Interpersonal skills

IX. Orientation
A. Definition
B. Overview
C. Induction training
1. Purpose
2. Content
3. Process
a. Time frame
b. Institutional perspectives
c. Targeting content
D. Job orientation
1. Match of employee background and orientation
2. Centralized or decentralized; standardized or individualized
3. Relationship to agency philosophy and purpose
4. Content
5. Conducted by area supervisor or designee
E. Adult education theory
1. Principles
2. Methods
F. Internships
1. Provides bridge
2. Guidelines
a. Preceptor:nurse ratio
b. Activity overview
c. Suggested time periods
3. Advantages
4. Four level example
G. Preceptor system
1. Characteristics
2. Example

X. Summary

CLASSROOM ACTIVITY: Recruitment and Selection for a Pediatric ICU staff nurse and/or a surgical intensive care staff nurse for the Over 70s unit at Podville Hospital.

The following activities incorporate aspects of chapter objectives 2 and 3. In addition, the activities will better prepare students for the roles of interviewee and interviewer.

Objective 2: Outline steps of a recruitment plan for attracting a suitable mix of newly graduated and more experienced nurses to your unit.

Objective 3: List content topics for a newspaper or journal advertisement to attract applicants for employment in your agency.

Time: The following activities may be divided into two class sessions.

Situation:

Openings for registered nurses exist in Podville Hospital's pediatric ICU unit and in the Over 70s surgical intensive care unit. See Figure 12.1 of this *Manual* for the structure of the pediatric unit, and Figure 13.1 for the structure of the Over 70s unit. Since Podville Hospital's administration practices decentralized nursing management, the pediatric selection committee is composed of the Divisional Director-Pediatrics, the Pediatric Nurse Clinician, and a pediatric ICU staff nurse. The over 70's selection committee is composed of the Divisional Director-Over 70s unit, Gerontology Nurse Clinician, and an Over 70s surgical intensive care staff nurse.

Activities

1. Through classroom discussion, determine additional parameters needed to further define position and position needs, e.g., special certification, experience, and educational qualifications; special needs given current staff nurse mix; availability and flexibility needs. (10 minutes)
2. Select ideas from the class for appropriate recruitment activities.
3. Solicit ideas from the class for an advertisement for each of the positions. The advertisements are to be placed in a local newspaper. Write the adds on the blackboard.

   (10-15 minutes for 2 + 3)
4. Select:

   Two groups of three students each are taken to a separate area and will be the applicants.

   A third group of three students are to be the Divisional Director - Pediatrics, the Pediatric Nurse Clinician, and the pediatric ICU staff nurse.

   A fourth group of three students are to be the Divisional Director-Over 70s unit, the Gerontology Nurse Clinician, and an Over 70s surgical intensive care staff nurse.

   The third and fourth groups come to the front of the classroom and elicit from the class (1) the questions that are to be asked during the interview, and (2) the way to set up the interview area.

   While the third and fourth groups are planning the interview, the faculty assigns roles to each of the applicants:

One applicant in each group is capable, experienced, meets the criteria identified by the class, but does not communicate. This applicant is to respond in polite, pleasant monosyllables, without volunteering information or explicating on anything.

One applicant in each group is to be a very verbal, aggressive, take-over kind of person who is overqualified in experience and education, and was asked to resign from her last position.

The third applicant in each group is underqualified in education and experience, but is an eager potentially capable person with excellent references. Her reason for applying for the position is so she "can grow."

Each applicant is to complete an "application" for the interviewers. The applicants are to present qualifications as defined by the class in the best light possible.

5. Choosing applicants for interviews:

   The faculty delivers the "applications" to the respective interviewers. Each group of interviewers, with class input, decide which of the three applicants they will interview. (5-10 minutes)

   Faculty: Students may decide to interview each of the three, or only one or two. Be prepared to respect their decision and proceed. It will not be surprising if they resist interviewing the third applicant. If that is the case, do allow the group to reconsider this decision after conducting the first one or two interviews.

6. Interviewing: (Time 10-15 minutes per interview)

   Students who are not part of the groups are instructed to note activities and communication techniques. Note both verbal and nonverbal examples. The Memo Capsule on page 246 of the text will be helpful in their critique.

   The interviewers call in (one at a time) the applicants to be interviewed. The interviewers pursue the formulated plan for the interview. The applicants play their respective roles.

7. Selection:

   The applicants are allowed to resume their place in class.

   The interviewers, with class input, summarize on the blackboard the applicants' educational and experiential backgrounds using the format of Table 13-1 of the text as a guide.

   A similar summary should also be made for the personal and/or unique characteristics that the group has identified.

   Guide the group to a unified decision for each position.

   Student decisions may include selection, or impasse, or decision to interview another, a decision to reopen the search, or a decision to "retrain" someone in house. This is a good time to tell the students the undiscovered "facts" about their applicants. The exercise will help students to learn both the value and limitations of the interview and selection process.

ASSIGNMENT: Writing an Ad

The activity will implement chapter objective 3.

Objective 3: List current topics for a newspaper or journal advertisement to attract applicants for employment in your agency.

Ask students to write a 55 word (or less) advertisement for a specific position at a facility with which they are familiar.

Criteria: The advertisements should include the four "Ps" of marketing. (See Memo Capsule on page 237 of text.)

GROUP PROJECT: Orientation to Podville Hospital's Pediatrics or Over 70s units

The project is suitable for generic BSN and experienced nurses.

Situation:
In a previous activity, students selected an applicant for a position as an ICU pediatrics staff nurse or a surgical intensive care staff nurse for the Over 70s unit.

Activities

Time: 30 minutes

1. Discuss and decide the approach to be used for pediatrics orientation or Over 70s unit orientation; e.g., Who is to conduct the program? Is a preceptor approach to be used? (5 minutes)

2. Divide class into four groups. Groups 1 and 2 are assigned the Pediatrics unit and Groups 3 and 4 are assigned the Over 70s unit.

   Groups 1 and 3 assignment: Induction

   List the induction content for assigned units that should be shared with each newly hired unit nurse. Which items should be shared in a "handbook"?

   Note: The content is to be in common throughout the hospital. Students may find Figure 13-4 of the text helpful.

   Groups 2 and 4 assignment: Position orientation

   Design a check list to be used to orient the newly selected Pediatric ICU staff nurse (Group 2), or the Over 70s Surgical Intensive care unit nurse (Group 4).

3. When both groups have completed their projects, have the group leaders share their products. Be sure to meld the induction and position orientation components for each unit to present a complete orientation program.

TEST QUESTIONS

KNOWLEDGE AND COMPREHENSION

True : False

T F 13.01. The single most effective nurse recruiter is a satisfied nurse employed at the facility.

T F 13.02. Indoctrination content of an orientation program is best individualized.

T F 13.03. The purpose of induction is to verify the readiness of the newly hired nurse to administer patient care.

T F 13.04. Most nurses use a rational multi-step process in searching for a position.

Multiple Choice

13.05. Recruitment is made easier if:
- a. a nursing personnel profile is completed
- b. a separate recruitment office is set up
- c. the personnel office does all of the recruiting
- d. all of above

13.06. The nurse recruiter needs:
- a. knowledge of the health agency philosophy, purpose, and program
- b. to project a positive, personable image
- c. to be knowledgeable regarding the types and numbers of area nursing graduates
- d. all of above

13.07. Before nurses are recruited:
- a. exit interviews have been used to resolve problems
- b. the number and type of staff needed for care are established
- c. determine the geographic region from which current nurse employees have come
- d. all of above

13.08. The value of exit interviews lies in:
- a. the accuracy of the information obtained
- b. its reflection of employee capabilities
- c. revealing sources of job dissatisfaction
- d. all of above

13.09. The four "Ps" of marketing are:
- a. product, place, promotion, and price.
- b. plan, people, placement, productivity.
- c. potential, pace, participation, patience.
- d. publicity, perception, persistence, power.

13.10. Which of the following should be included when marketing a position?
- a. promotion of opportunities
- b. high quality care
- c. inservice education opportunities
- d. all of above

13.11. In a decentralized agency who will preferably interview an applicant?
- a. nurse administrator
- b. immediate supervisor of position
- c. personnel officer
- d. committee of staff nurses
- e. a and c

13.12. To compare several qualified applicants for one position, the manager will:
- a. compare educational backgrounds
- b. take notes during interviews
- c. compare experience backgrounds
- d. choose the applicant about whom s/he feels best
- e. a and c

13.13. The induction portion of orientation should include:
  a. payday, parking and eating facilities.
  b. self-evaluation on a check list.
  c. skills verification.
  d. all of above

13.14. For maximum usefulness an orientation handbook will:
  a. cross-index all topics
  b. contain employee responsibilities
  c. include agency obligations
  d. all of above

13.15. When is the new employee most likely to adopt the organization's view point?
  a. when comfortable in new position
  b. during induction
  c. while working with a preceptor
  d. after the skills check list is completed

13.16. Which of the following are characteristics of a preceptor approach to orientation?
  a. four progressive level of performance are identified for the orientee
  b. an experienced nurse is paired and scheduled with the orientee
  c. the orientation experience includes a rotation to several departments
  d. all of above

APPLICATION, ANALYSIS, AND/OR SYNTHESIS

Multiple Choice

13.17. Unit manager Ms. On Theball is gathering information for a nursing personnel profile for her unit. She will include:
  1. average rate of nurse staff absenteeism by unit and job classification
  2. annual nursing staff turnover rate by unit and job classification
  3. a comprehensive recruitment plan
  4. percentage of nurses by educational background and job classification
  a. 1, 2
  b. 2, 3
  c. 1, 2, 4
  d. all of above

13.18. Nurse recruiter Wiseone has completed a comprehensive nursing personnel profile. Ms. Wiseone will first:
  a. share information to inquirers at a career day to see what appeals to them
  b. share information with nursing administration for potential correction/improvement
  c. convey information in attractive succinct brochures
  d. caution applicants regarding the limitations of the agency as noted in the profile

13.19. Nurse recruiter Wiseone is to secure applications for a unit nurse manager. Which of the following journals would be the most likely to reach qualified potential applicants?
  a. *RN*
  b. *Journal of Nursing Administration*
  c. *Nurse Educator*
  d. *Nursing Research*

13.20. You are a nurse manager and want the orientation program to be updated to better prepare nurses to work on the various units. You will:
  a. ask the inservice director to update the orientation program
  b. ask the personnel department to update the orientation program
  c. select nurses from the units to recommend revision
  d. appoint nurse managers to a committee to revise the orientation program

13.21. Job orientation for the newly hired ICU pediatric staff nurse is best supervised by the:
  a. inservice director
  b. pediatric clinician
  c. immediate supervisor
  d. personnel office

13.22. Which of the following best demonstrates the application of adult education theory in an orientation program?
   a. The new nurse identifies the skills she would like demonstrated.
   b. The head nurse gives the new nurse a patient care assignment.
   c. The inservice educator prepares and presents an orientation class.
   d. The inservice educator demonstrated job required skills.

Matching: The recruitment committee desires to project various images for different positions. Match the brochure description to the most likely applicant market it will attract.

	Market/Image	Description
____	13.23. Nursing students for summer OR internship program	a. light gray parchment paper with bold black classic print
____	13.24. Staff who value caring	b. bright green heavy paper picturing a patient having a scan
____	13.25. Staff with a high priority on monetary values	c. rich pale blue paper picturing a nurse talking with an elderly patient
____	13.26. Quiet, stable, conservative	d. slick red paper with silver printed salary schedules

ANSWERS	TEXT REFERENCE
13.01. T	p. 241
13.02. F	p. 249
13.03. F	p. 249
13.04. F	p. 242
13.05. a	p. 236
13.06. d	p. 2235, 236
13.07. d	p. 236
13.08. c	p. 236, 237
13.09. a	p. 237
13.10. d	p. 237, 240
13.11. b	p. 244
13.12. e	p. 247
13.13. a	p. 249
13.14. d	p. 249
13.15. b	p. 249
13.16. b	p. 255
13.17. c	p. 236
13.18 b	p. 236
13.19. b	p. 239
13.20. c	p. 253
13.21. c	p. 253
13.22. a	p. 253, 254
13.23. b	p. 240
13.24. c	p. 240
13.25. d	p. 240
13.26. a	p. 240

CHAPTER

14

Scheduling

Scheduling incorporates all of the staffing activities discussed to this point. The results of scheduling impact the quality and type of care that can be given and impact staff productivity and morale. The activities presented for this chapter will give students the opportunity to experience the multiple factors that must be included when creating a staffing schedule, and the complexity of the task.

KEY TERMS

cyclical scheduling
float pool
scheduling
shiftwork
staff leveling
staffing
supplemental agency

OUTLINE

I. Scheduling overview
   A. Staffing defined
   B. Scheduling defined
   C. Steps
   D. Importance

II. Scheduling policies
   A. List of needed policies
   B. Issues
      1. Scheduling clerk
      2. Governmental regulations
      3. Rotation practices
      4. Posting
      5. Week ends and shifts
      6. "First" day of week
      7. Days off

III. Scheduling responsibility

IV. Cyclical scheduling
   A. Described
   B. Principles for effective cyclical scheduling

V. Causes of overstaffing
   A. Patient census variations
   B. Staffing for maximum census
   C. Reasons for overstaffing

VI. Controlled variable staffing
   A. Defined
   B. Minimum staffing level

1. Example
2. Varying numbers of staff
3. Varying shift times

C. Obtaining additional personnel
1. Temporary reassignment
2. Float pools
3. Stand-by, on-call
4. Supplemental nursing agency
5. Nurse registry

D. Reasons for using variable staffing
1. Cost containment
2. Staff leveling

VII. Shiftwork
A. Defined
B. Personal toll
C. Recommendations

VIII. Summary

CLASSROOM ACTIVITIES: Scheduling for Podville Hospital

The following activities incorporate chapter objectives 1 and 2.

Objective 1: Design a cyclical staffing schedule for all nursing service personnel on your unit that will provide adequate numbers of each category of personnel on each shift for forecasted numbers and types of patients.

Objective 2: Write policies to guide employees in reporting sick time and requesting special time off to support the cyclical staffing schedule for your unit.

Time: 2 class periods

Activities

Divide class into small groups. Groups may choose to schedule staff for the Pediatrics unit of Podville Hospital (Figure 12.1), or the Over 70s unit (Figure 13.1).

1. Each group is to follow the steps needed for staffing.
   - Determine hours of maximum and minimum workload.
   - Determine types of workers needed (RN, LPN, Assistant, level and experience of RNs).
   - Establish policies applicable to scheduling.
   - Identify "shifts" to be used.
   - Determine numbers and types of staff needed for minimum, average, and maximum census for 24 hour coverage.
2. Design a cyclical staffing schedule to cover the minimum census with options for dealing with understaffing situations.
3. Who will be responsible for implementing the options for adjusting staffing on a shift-by-shift basis?

   How will the options for adjusting staffing on a shift-by-shift basis be implemented?

DISCUSSION: Minimizing Negatives of Shift Rotation

Question: When designing a cyclical staffing pattern, what can be done to minimize the negative effects of shift rotations?

See Memo Capsule on page 266 of text for possible responses.

TEST QUESTIONS

KNOWLEDGE AND COMPREHENSION

True : False

T F 14.01. Scheduling and staffing are the same thing.

T F 14.02. The staff will perceive the "scheduler" as a manager.

T F 14.03. Labor contracts contain policies which pertain to scheduling.

T F 14.04. A policy to schedule two days off a week supports scheduling flexibility.

T F 14.05. Personnel cost containment requires use of some form of variable staffing.

T F 14.06. Research has demonstrated that rapid shift turnover has little effect on work efficiency.

Multiple Choice

14.07. Scheduling impacts:
- a. employee productivity
- b. employee morale
- c. patient care quality
- d. all of above

14.08. Scheduling policies need to include:
- a. posting time
- b. number of paid holidays per year
- c. start of work week
- d. all of above

14.09. Reduction of invested time in scheduling can best be achieved by:
- a. utilizing cyclical scheduling
- b. utilizing unit managers to do scheduling
- c. disallowing personal requests for days off
- d. establishing float nurse pools

14.10. Variable staffing requires:
- a. a minimum staff base
- b. all RN staffing
- c. a modular delivery system
- d. all of above

14.11. A(n) advantage(s) of 12-hour shifts include(s):
- a. improved communication between shifts
- b. extended time for leisure and social activities
- c. reduction of overtime and absenteeism
- d. all of above

14.12. The chief disadvantage of 10- and 12-hour shifts over 8-hour shifts is:
- a. task assignment
- b. staff fatigue
- c. accountability
- d. increase in sick time

14.13. Overstaffing occurs because of:
- a. frequent variations in patient care needs
- b. unpredictable variations in patient census
- c. staffing for maximum census
- d. all of above

14.14. The use of frequent "pulling" of personnel from one unit to another to cover changing patient census will:
a. increase staff growth
b. cause staff anxiety
c. promote continuity of care
d. all of above

14.15. Which of the following is characteristic of a supplemental staff agency?
a. it is a state licensed referral agency
b. it employs nurses and assigns them to facilities on a contractual basis
c. functions as an internal float pool
d. all of above

APPLICATION, ANALYSIS, AND/OR SYNTHESIS

Multiple Choice

14.16. The nurse manager is reviewing scheduling practices for her unit with the intent of revising the schedules. In what order will she do the following?
1. determine on/off pattern
2. determine workload
3. check for errors
4. identify budgeted and filled positions
5. analyze unit's work flow
a. 1,2,3,4,5
b. 4,1,3,2,5
c. 5,2,4,1,3
d. 2,4,5,1,3

14.17. Podville Hospital's Over 70s unit staff is implementing a new cyclical schedule. Which of the following should be an outcome?
a. increased need to draw upon the float pool
b. promotion of continuity of care and teamwork
c. concentration of best qualified nurses during active day hours
d. all of above

14.18. Nurse Administrator Wiseone notes that newer nurse manager Iam Shigh is repeatedly overstaffing her unit. Which of the following actions on the part of Nurse Administrator Wiseone has the greatest potential for good long-term resolution?
a. Nurse Administrator Wiseone takes over the scheduling of Iam Shigh's unit
b. Nurse Administrator Wiseone delegates the scheduling of Iam Shigh's unit to the personnel office
c. Nurse Administrator Wiseone meets with Iam Shigh to review the scheduling pattern
d. Nurse Administrator Wiseone places Iam Shigh on probation as a nurse manager

14.19. Since the Podville Hospital Over 70s unit has implemented cyclical scheduling the patients frequently complain about evening care. Which of the following will assist the unit manager in problem resolution?
a. review the way in which nursing staff is used throughout the 24 hour day
b. revise the sick leave and personal request policies
c. copy the staffing pattern of another unit which is not experiencing this problem
d. request an additional nursing position for the evening shift

ANSWERS	TEXT REFERENCE
14.01. F	p. 258
14.02. T	p. 260
14.03. T	p. 260
14.04. F	p. 260
14.05. T	p. 265
14.06. F	p. 266
14.07. d	p. 258
14.08. d	p. 259, 260
14.09. a	p. 261
14.10. a	p. 263
14.11. d	p. 264
14.12. b	p. 264
14.13. d	p. 261-263
14.14. b	p. 264
14.15. b	p. 265
14.16. c	p. 258, 259
14.17. b	p. 261
14.18. c	p. 262
14.19. a	p. 261

CHAPTER

15

Patient Classification and Acuity Systems

Nursing staff and nursing managers have both discovered a need to staff according to actual patient care needs. The task of reducing patient care needs to quantifiable data is a challenge that has been met through several different approaches. Various ways of determining patient care needs, and devising a classification system upon which to base staffing are presented in this chapter.

KEY TERMS

care intensity
content validity
criterion based validity
face validity
factor system
Medisgroups
nursing intensity
patient classification system
P.I.N.I.
prospective payment
prototype system
reliability
retrospective payment
validity

OUTLINE

I. Introduction
  A. Need for balanced workload and staffing
  B. Impact of over and under staffing

II. Measuring nursing workload
  A. Evolutionary perspective
    1. Patient census
    2. Patient condition
      a. Patient diagnosis
      b. Additional variables
    3. Goal
  B. Components of nursing workload
    1. Forecasting workload
    2. Review of past patterns
  C. Purpose of patient classification systems
    1. Defined
    2. Purpose
    3. Components
  D. Types of patient classification systems

1. Prototype
   a. Description
   b. Methodology
2. Factor
   a. Description
   b. Methodology

E. Factor evaluation system
   1. Care descriptor
   2. Levels of care intensity
      a. Time quantification per descriptor
      b. Examples

F. Prototype evaluation system
   1. Category examples given

III. Designing a patient classification system
   A. Accuracy versus time savings
   B. Tailor to setting

IV. Validity and reliability of classification tool
   A. Validity defined
      1. Face validity
      2. Content validity
      3. Criterion-based validity
   B. Reliability defined

V. Nursing time standards
   A. Methods
      1. Estimating
      2. Historical averaging
      3. Time logging
      4. Work sampling
      5. Industry standards
      6. Time and motion studies
   B. Determining professional and nonprofessional personnel mix
      1. Percentage examples given
      2. Full-time to part-time ratios given

VI. Diagnostic related groups
   A. History
   B. Retrospective payment system
      1. DRG categories
      2. Cost containment
      3. Concerns
      4. Research findings
      5. Nursing costs
      6. Care intensity

VII. Severity of illness measures
   A. Purpose
   B. Common measures
      1. Computerized severity of illness index
      2. Disease staging
      3. Medical illness severity grouping system

VIII. Nursing intensity measures
   A. Defined
   B. Four dimensions
      1. Illness severity
      2. Patient dependency
      3. Nursing care complexity
      4. Time

VIII. Summary

CLASS DISCUSSION: Measuring Nursing Workload

Designate a unit of a facility with which students are familiar.

Time: 15 minutes

Question: If the facility were to designate charges for actual nursing services rather than a room rate, what factors would need to be included. Use text pages 270, 271 as a resource.

Responses should include:
- medical diagnosis
- severity of illness
- complexity of care
- general physical condition
- social-psychological status
- age
- sex
- type of staff and expertise level
- projected service use
- physical facilities

GROUP PROJECT: Prototype Patient Classification System

The following activity implements a portion of chapter objective 1: "Explain the difference between a prototype and a factor type patient classification system."

Time: 45 minutes

Situation: The Nurse Unit Manager for Podville Hospital's Over 70s unit is exploring new patient classification systems. The staff are accustomed to thinking of patients as needing different levels of care; therefore, the unit manager first explores a prototype approach to patient classification. The services that the Over 70s unit provides for persons over 70 years of age are surgical intensive care, medical intensive care, general medical-surgical care, a short-term stay unit for 9:00 am to 9:00 pm, and with respite care by reservation from 9:00 pm to 9:00 am.

Activities

1. Divide class into smaller groups.
2. Each group is to identify five categories into which the Over 70s unit patients would be classified. (25 minutes)
3. Have groups share their products with entire class. (10 minutes)
4. Draw from the class the likely limitations of applying the categories.
5. What are advantages of using this type of system? (10 minutes)

GROUP PROJECT: Long Term Care Resident Classification System

The project incorporates chapter objectives 2 and 3.

Objective 2: Explain the difference between a task-based and an acuity-based patient classification system.

Objective 3: List five care descriptors that are commonly used in a factor-type patient classification system.

Situation: You are the nursing administrator of a long term care unit. The structure of the facility is composed of three wings. Each wing offers a broadly designated focus:

Unit 1: provides services for residents needing self-care services but who do not need special nursing services beyond medications or dietary supplements.

Unit 2: provides services for residents with long term illnesses and persons needing short term skilled nursing needs.

Unit 3: provides services for persons with psychological and self-care needs who may or may not have additional medical needs.

Divide class into three groups. Each group is assigned one unit.

Assignment

Identify 8-10 task-based factors for the designated population which could be used in developing a facility-wide resident care classification system.

HOMEWORK ASSIGNMENT: Care descriptors for Podville Hospital's Over 70s unit

In the following activities, students apply chapter objective 3.

Objective 3: List five care descriptors that are commonly used in a factor-type patient classification system.

Situation: The unit manager and staff for Podville Hospital's Over 70s unit decide that the categories they identified are inadequate for predicting needed nursing care, and decide to design a factor-type patient classification system. Again, the services provided by the Over 70s unit are for persons over 70 years of age and include surgical intensive care, medical intensive care, general medical-surgical care, a short-term stay unit from 9:00 am to 9:00 pm, and respite care 9:00 pm to 9:00 am by reservation.

Assignment

1. Identify care descriptors applicable to all of the Over 70s unit patients.

   Identify additional care descriptors applicable to only one or two of the services.

Try to limit descriptors to 10 - 15 and at the same time promote inclusivity. See text pages 7-9 and Figure 15-3 as a resource.

Criteria: Descriptors should include considerations of patient needs because of aging as well as descriptors specific to the services.

2. Choose one of the descriptors identified above that applies to all services. Specify four levels of the descriptor. Assign point values to each of these levels. Use Memo Capsule page 272 of text as a resource.

CLASS ACTIVITY: Interrater Reliability

Objective 5 is met in the following activity.

Objective 5: Describe one method for determining interrater reliability of the patient-classification tool that is used in your health agency.

1. Write task based factors identified by the students in the Long Term Resident Classification System activity (above) on the blackboard or on an overhead.

2. Read the following case study to the class.
    - Admitted from home via medical transport an 84 year old 90 pound married female.
    - Family states she is dependent for all ADLs.
    - Lacks mobility related to impaired mental function and absent left hip joint.
    - Unable to feed self and family reports she sometimes forgets how to swallow.
    - She arrived with indwelling catheter. Urine cloudy and scant with strong odor.
    - Family states they give her an enema every third day.
    - Is on major tranquilizer to control behavior. family states that she can be surprisingly strong and combative.
3. A sk students to each classify the patient using the factors on the blackboard.
4. Poll students as to the factors they used.
5. Note similarities and differences and discuss in light of interrater reliability.
6. What might be done to improve interrater reliability?

    Text pages 274 and 275 may be used as a reference. Both validity and reliability may need to be addressed.

TEST QUESTIONS

KNOWLEDGE AND COMPREHENSION

True : False

T F 15.01. The amount of nursing resources required by a patient in a given DRG is relatively constant throughout a patient's hospitalization.

T F 15.02. Research demonstrates that patients in the same DRG show comparable severity levels in different hospitals.

Multiple Choice

15.03. Nursing personnel dissatisfaction and excessive turnover are outcomes of:
a. understaffing
b. overstaffing
c. both over and under staffing

15.04. The most accurate way to predict nursing costs is to utilize a system based upon:
a. quantity and quality of care
b. patient diagnoses
c. average patient census
d. DRGs

15.05. Which of the following is needed to achieve maximum cost-effective personnel allocation?
a. determine number of personnel needed
b. determine type of personnel needed
c. predetermine standards of care
d. all of above

15.06. The purpose(s) of patient classification systems is(are) to:
a. implement DRGs cost-effectively
b. assess patient: nursing needs
c. minimize DRG outliers
d. all of above

15.07. In a factor type patient classification system, point values assigned to descriptors indicate:
a. types of personnel needed
b. rank order of needs
c. standard time required for elements of care
d. all of above

15.08. A valid patient classification system implemented at one facility:
a. needs to be tailored if used at another facility
b. can be readily transferred to another facility of the same kind but not different kinds of facilities
c. can be transferred to other facilities regardless of type
d. is institutionally specific and is best not used in another facility

APPLICATION, ANALYSIS, AND/OR SYNTHESIS

Multiple Choice

15.09. Podville Hospital's Over 70s nurse unit manager wants to implement a more effective patient classification system and decides to use a factor system. The nurse unit manager will first identify:

a. four or five categories reflecting degree of patient dependency
b. care descriptors
c. nursing tasks
d. standards of performance

15.10. Which of the following would be descriptors that could be used in designing a patient care system for Podville Hospital's Over 70s unit?

a. activities of daily living, mobility
b. patient length of stay compared to average length of stay
c. moderate and extensive care
d. all of above

15.11. Which of the following represents content validity for point values assigned to activities of daily living (ADL) criteria developed for the Over 70s unit of Podville Hospital?

a. the points appear to measure weighted time it takes nurses to perform ADLs
b. the long and short versions of the patient classification system produce the same assessment
c. the point values are twice as much for bathing the patient as for self-bathing and it takes the nurse twice as long to bath a patient as to guide the patient in self-bathing
d. total ADL time is accounted for in the point values

15.12. Which of the following activities represents interrater reliability as the new patient classification system is applied to the Over 70s unit in Podville Hospital?

a. needed nursing care is accurately predicted by the unit manager
b. the staff nurse and the unit manager each assign the patient the same classification level
c. nursing care standards can be developed for each of the identified items
d. the applied system predicts nursing care needs within a + or - ten percent

Matching: Match the terms to the descriptions by placing the appropriate letter in the space provided. A term will be used more than once

Descriptions

___ 15.13. The East coast Visiting Nurse Association identified five categories for a rehabilitation patient classification system.

___ 5.14. Staff nurses of the unit reviewed the criteria and agreed that the criteria looked appropriate.

___ 15.15. The Resident classification system designed for Unit 1 of the long-term care facility well rep resented the types of care needed.

___ 15.16. The consultant randomly observes and records nursing personnel activities.

___ 15.17. The hospital received a daily dollar amount to cover nursing, ancillary and hospital services and a separate payment for each service not covered.

___ 15.18. The hospital will be paid X amount for DRG 336.

___ 15.19. Patient X is classified by the computer into one of five groups using key findings.

___ 15.20. P.I.N.I.

___ 15.21. Patient X will need 15 minutes of a clinical nurse specialist care, 20 minutes of RN care, and 1.5 hours of nursing assistant care.

Terms

a. content validity

b. face validity

c. Medisgroups

d. nursing intensity measures

e. prospective system

f. prototype system

g. retrospective system

h. work sampling

ANSWERS	TEXT REFERENCE
15.01. F	p. 278
15.02. F	p. 278
15.03. c	p. 270
15.04. a	p. 270
15.05. d	p. 270
15.06. b	p. 271
15.07. c	p. 271, 272
15.08. d	p. 271
15.09. b	p. 272
15.10. a	p. 272
15.11. c	p. 274
15.12. b	p. 275
15.13. f	p. 273
15.14. b	p. 274
15.15. a	p. 274
15.16. h	p. 275
15.17. g	p. 277
15.18. e	p. 277
15.19. c	p. 279
15.20. d	p. 279, 280
15.21. d	p. 279, 280

CHAPTER

16

Absenteeism

Maintaining adequate staffing in times of limited resources, both economic and human, is a challenge to today's nurse manager. One place "additional" staffing may be found is in the reduction of the staff absentee rate. A look at why staff are absent, which of the staff are absent, and patterns of absence can help the nurse manager identify changes in unit management which will promote a decrease in the staff absentee rate and thus increase availability of staff for work.

OUTLINE

I. Introduction
   A. Rationale for importance
   B. Definition
   C. Historical trends

II. Computing absenteeism
   A. Time lost percentage
   B. Absence frequency rate
   C. Absentee patterns

III. Effects of absenteeism
   A. Economic costs
   B. Inefficiencies
   C. Decreased employee morale
   D. Increase staffing by reducing absenteeism

IV. Types of absenteeism
   A. Unavoidable
   B. Voluntary

V. Pattern of absenteeism
   A. Frequency
   B. Work time loss patterns
   C. Demographic variables
   D. "Stringing" phenomenon

VI. Factors contributing to absenteeism
   A. Study findings
      1. Theories of absence
         a. Economic
         b. Psychological
         c. Sociologic
         d. Jurisprudential
         e. Disability
      2. Correlation between overtime and absence
      3. Proximity of home to work
      4. Size of work groups
      5. Types of illnesses
      6. Correlation between absenteeism rates and accident rates
   B. Emotional causes for absenteeism
      1. Relationship to personality characteristics
      2. Relationship to self-concept
      3. Relationship to job dissatisfaction
   C. Weak work ethic
   D. Poor personnel policies

VII. Methods of reducing absenteeism
   A. Accurate records
   B. Counseling re excessive absences
   C. Formal "call in" procedure
   D. Visiting nurses
   E. Free health care
   F. Safety and accident program
   G. Improve work milieu
      1. Democratic management practices
      2. Flexible scheduling
   I. Incentive plans
   J. Child care
   K. Disciplinary measures

VIII. Summary

DISCUSSION IDEA: Voluntary, involuntary absences

The discussion pertains to chapter objectives 2 and 3.

Objective 2: Interview three coworkers to determine their usual reason(s) for absenteeism.

Objective 3: Suggest one managerial intervention to minimize each cause cited for absenteeism by your three coworkers.

Situation: The Podville Hospital Over 70s unit is experiencing a 5% absence rate of its nursing staff.

Elicit from students possible reasons for absences.

Identify which of these reasons are voluntary and which are involuntary.

What might be done to reduce the absence rate? Consider suggestions in the text and/or student ideas.

GROUP ACTIVITY: Absenteeism

Chapter objectives 2 and 3 can be translated into this group activity.

Objective 2: Interview three coworkers to determine their usual reason(s) for absenteeism.

Objective 3: Suggest one managerial intervention to minimize each cause cited for absenteeism by your three coworkers.

Time: 25 minutes plus discussion time

Activities

Divide class into smaller groups.

Each group is to:

- identify three reasons why they have been absent from work (or school).
- state a managerial intervention to minimize each of the causes of the absence.

Reconvene class

- list absence reasons on blackboard
- have each group share one managerial intervention strategy, relating the intervention to the absence reason.

GROUP PROJECT: An incentive plan to reduce absenteeism

Designing an incentive plan is a management intervention that implements a portion of chapter objective 3: "Suggest one managerial intervention to minimize each cause cited for absenteeism by your three coworkers."

Time: 30 minutes plus discussion of plans

Situation: The Podville Hospital Over 70s unit is experiencing a 5% absence rate of its nursing staff. The Over 70s unit manager wants to design an incentive plan that maximizes recognition, has long, medium, and short range perspectives, has a low economic impact, and does not use planned absence days as a reward. The group represents an Over 70s unit staff committee who will make recommendations to the unit manager.

Activities

1. Create an incentive plan which will reward staff attendance.

   Include incentives for different periods of time, i.e., quarterly, six months, annually.

   Do try to avoid punishing or rewarding through peers. Do target individual staff behavior.

2. As a class, discuss the ideas of the groups. Critique the ideas as to their overall appeal, costs, and amount of managerial time each would require to implement.

3. Have class select "the best" incentive approach for each time period.

TEST QUESTIONS

KNOWLEDGE AND COMPREHENSION

True : False

T F 16.01. The first step in reducing absenteeism is to keep accurate records of employee absenteeism.

T F 16.02. Home visits by a nurse to sick employees improved employee attendance rates.

T F 16.03. Twelve hour schedules increased employee absence.

T F 16.04. Incentive programs have proven ineffective in reducing employee absenteeism.

Completion

_____ 16.05. According to data of the Bureau of National Affairs, the annual absenteeism rates for health care workers is ? days per year.

Multiple Choice

16.06. Nurse Unit Manager Dogood needs more staff to cover the unit and requests an absenteeism profile of the unit staff. The usefulness of this request lies in the fact that:
a. identification of employees who are frequently absent can lead to corrective actions
b. twenty percent of the employees are reported to be responsible for 80% of the absences
c. a 4% loss of hours is experienced in medical organizations
d. all of above

16.07. Outcomes of a high absenteeism rate include:
a. increased staffing costs
b. decreased employee morale
c. greater inefficiencies and more errors
d. all of above

16.08. Implementation of a combined leave benefit system resulted in:
a. greater use of unscheduled days off
b. more use of extended illness days off
c. reduction in overtime hours
d. need for closer supervision of replacement workers

16.09. On-site sick and well child care facilities:
a. reduce employee absenteeism
b. improve employee productivity
c. have a negative cost:benefit ratio
d. a and b
e. a and c

APPLICATION, ANALYSIS, AND/OR SYNTHESIS

Multiple Choice

16.10. Which of the following potential employee profiles would most likely have a lower absenteeism rate?
  a. applicant Urswell reports no absences in his last job of two years
  b. applicant Outhere states that her willingness to commute a considerable distance demonstrates how much she wants the job
  c. applicant ReSourceful says that she will be able to get a ride to the expressway where she will use public transportation to reach the facility
  d. the profiles do not present significant differences as they relate to absenteeism

16.11. Nurse Unit Manager Dogood is reviewing staffing patterns with the purpose of decreasing the high absenteeism rate among newer nursing staff. Which of the following staffing proposals would most likely contribute to less absenteeism?
  a. institute modular staffing with the pairing of a new RN or nursing assistant with a senior nurse
  b. implement paid on-call system for times of additional staff need
  c. recommendation of a policy that staff must obtain coverage for their own absences
  d. promote a staffing ratio adequate for average nursing care demands which is greater than the minimum staffing ratio in use

16.12. Nurse Unit Manager Dogood is concerned with the high incidence of employee tardiness and a high accident rate. Again Nurse Unit Manager Dogood examines the absentee patterns. The examination of the absentee patterns is:
  a. inappropriate as absenteeism, tardiness, and accidents are separate issues
  b. useful as there is a high correlation in absentee, tardy, and accident occurrence for the same employee
  c. not relevant as accident rates pertain to inattentiveness, inappropriate use of equipment, or lack of knowledge
  d. useful as a greater incidence of tardiness occurs when absentee rates are higher

16.13. Nurse Unit Manager Dogood knows that low self-concept correlates positively with high absentee patterns. Which of the following will Ms. Dogood promote to increase employee self-concept?
  a. a practice of a home nursing visit by facility personnel on an employee's third absent day
  b. facilitate staff identification of goals to be pursued in conjunction with position
  c. provide empathy to the absent employee to demonstrate consideration and support
  d. all of above

16.14. Nurse Unit Manager Dogood notices that a staff nurse has an absence rate of 4.8 per cent. Ms. Dogood should:
  a. compliment the staff nurse for her good work record.
  b. fire the staff nurse.
  c. counsel the staff nurse regarding her absences.
  d. do nothing at this time and continue to monitor absences.

ANSWERS	TEXT REFERENCE
16.01. T	p. 287
16.02. T	p. 287
16.03. F	p. 288
16.04. F	p. 288
16.05. 7	p. 283
16.06. d	p. 284
16.07. d	p. 284
16.08. c	p. 288
16.09. d	p. 286, 289
16.10. a	p. 285
16.11. a	p. 285, 286
16.12. b	p. 286
16.13. b	p. 286
16.14. c	p. 287

CHAPTER

17

Employee Turnover

As the nurse manager considers turnover rates, the challenges are to determine the optimum turnover rate, identify reasons for turnover, and evaluate every aspect of staffing to remedy problem areas. The chapter provides ideas to help nurse managers meet the challenges of bringing turnover rates into the optimum range. The group activities provide opportunity for students to practice application of these ideas.

KEY TERMS

correlational studies
exit interviews
involuntary turnover
role ambiguity
role conflict
role dissensus
turnover
voluntary turnover

OUTLINE

- I. Introduction
  - A. Definition of turnover
  - B. Use of turnover rates
  - C. Voluntary and involuntary turnover
- II. Computation of turnover rate
  - A. Formula
  - B. Examples of turnover rates
- III. Costs of personnel turnover
  - A. Financial costs
    1. Direct costs
    2. Indirect costs
    3. Research findings
  - B. Staff costs
    1. Lower morale
    2. Overstaffing for coverage
    3. Overburdening staff
    4. Strained interpersonal relationships
    5. Deterioration of patient care
  - C. Institutional costs
- IV. Optimum turnover rate
- V. Causes of avoidable turnover
  - A. Mismatch of institutional and employee needs
  - B. Poor respect accorded nurses
  - C. Dissatisfaction with role

D. Inadequate role definition
   1. Role conflict
   2. Role ambiguity
   3. Role dissensus
E. Education: practice disparity
F. Work schedule expectancies
G. Bureaucratic structures
H. Job dissatisfiers
I. Long-term ancillary staff power
J. Psychological characteristics

VI. Identifying causes of turnover
   A. Correlational studies
   B. Exit interviews
      1. Purposes
         a. Salvage employees
         b. Identify problems
      2. Conduct
      3. Example of results
   C. Post-termination polls
      1. Method
      2. Objectivity
   D. Attitude surveys
      1. Leavers and stayers
   E. Employee health and welfare committee
      1. Representation
      2. Purpose

VII. Methods for reducing turnover
   A. Revision of each staffing step
   B. Presentation of both positive and negative aspects
   C. Preemployment tour of unit
   D. Individualizing orientation
   E. Decrease education:practice disparity
   F. Stress reduction program
   G. Adjustment of assignment size
   H. Use of "nurse extenders"
   I. Match supervision needs to supervision practices
   J. Promote job satisfiers
   K. Improve performance evaluation
   L. Tailor interventions to longevity patterns
   M. Improvement in both personal and economic rewards
   N. Improvement in communication practices of entire health team
   O. Participative management
   P. Greater variety and flexibility of work schedules

VIII. Summary

GROUP PROJECT: Optimum turnover rate

The following activities practice chapter objective 1: "Compute turnover rates for RNs, LPNs, and aides in your nursing unit."

Time: 25 minutes

Situation: The text points out that some turnover is desirable to stimulate new ideas especially for problem solving. Ask students to recall how they chose to staff the Podville Hospital unit(s). Assign students to the same groups used for staffing activities presented in Chapters 12 and 13.

Activities

1. Given the staffing patterns identified by the students, state the number of staff of each category type who would optimally be replaced annually.
2. Once students have decided what would be desirable staff replacement, compute the overall nursing staff turnover rate. See text p. 293 for how to compute an annual turnover rate.
3. If the annual turnover rate is less than 5 percent or greater than 10 percent, the students are to change the recommendations of number 1 above to adjust the target turnover rate to the desired 5 to 10 percent range.

   What changes are recommended?
4. In the adjustment for achieving an optimum annual turnover rate, list policies, and/or practices that might need to be addressed? What changes are recommended?

GROUP PROJECT: Turnover and staff replacement analysis

This activity will guide students to meet and exceed chapter objectives 2.

Objective 2: List three costs involved in replacing a nurse who resigns from a position in your agency.

Time: 1 class period

Preparation: Reproduce Figure 17.1 at the end of this *Manual* for each group.

Introduction

Students profit by thinking through a problem in a comprehensive manner rather than just focusing on the obvious. Students are guided to think through the multiplicity of items that impact turnover rates and staff replacement. Figure 17.1. will guide student thinking utilizing familiar categories common to quality improvement analyses. The use of the categories beyond quality improvement activities has value in addition to the mechanics and learning that pertain to turnover issue. First-level nurse managers who need to add knowledge and understanding will find the activity very useful.

Staff turnover and replacement costs are obvious, hidden, and subtle. Staff turnover and replacement costs engulf human, facility, and economic resources. Staff replacement activities have structural, process, and outcome components.

Each of the above entities is to be considered in the project.

Situation

The Podville community long-term care facility is experiencing a long-term high annual turnover rate of its nursing staff. Administration would like to get at the heart of the turnover problems in contrast to using "quick-fix band-aide" solutions and has asked nursing management to succinctly present a comprehensive list of items which should be reviewed.

Activities

1. Using Figure 17.1, list items in each section which need to be reviewed to identify potential problem areas which are contributing to the high turnover rate and related staff replacement needs.

   To help you think of items:

   - List activities requiring dollar outlay ($-Process)
   - List items utilizing staff/management time (Human-Process)
   - List types of human expertise needed (Human-Structure)
   - State desired outcomes
     - outcomes that pertain to budget ($-Outcome)
     - outcomes pertaining to staffing levels and turnover rates (Human-Outcome)

   Note the examples which are included in Figure 17.1.

2. Most likely the group has been able to identify items which are more obvious. With just a little more thought, what might be some rather subtle entities that should also be considered? An example might be the attitude of senior nursing assistants toward new, inexperienced nursing assistants. Add these items to Figure 17.1.

Follow-up

Reconvene class and discuss the items the groups have identified.

When applied to a real situation, the use of Figure 19.1 will help to identify problem areas. The problem areas become apparent as there may be a preponderance of items or conversely no items in a particular section of the grid. For example, if desired outcomes or goals have not been carefully formulated, they may be unattainable, unrealistic, ambiguous, or nonexistent.

TEST QUESTIONS

KNOWLEDGE AND COMPREHENSION

True : False

T F 17.01. Nursing turnover rates are higher than are turnover rates in other industries.

T F 17.02. Turnover rates are computed using the average number of full time nursing positions.

T F 17.03. Creative or innovative nurses are less likely to quit positions in an agency practicing participative management

T F 17.04. A discrepancy between expected and experienced work schedules relates to intent to resign.

T F 17.05. An RN survey indicated a significant correlation between perceived work overload and intent to resign.

T F 17.06. Studies show that RN job satisfaction was increased when supervisors were older.

T F 17.07. The nurse manager will be most successful with all levels of personnel is s/he is consistent in management style.

Multiple Choice

17.08. Excessive turnover rates lead to which of the following?
  a. lower employee morale
  b. ineffective teamwork
  c. inability to grow staff for advanced positions
  d. all of above

17.09. Nurse Manager Upncomer is reviewing unit nursing staff turnover. To achieve an optimal turnover rate she has set which of the following as an annual turnover rate goal?
  a. 0 - 5%
  b. 5 - 10%
  c. 10 - 15%
  d. 15 - 20%

Matching: Match the turnover cost item to the type of cost by placing the correct letter in the space provided.

Examples of Turnover Costs	Types of Costs
____ 17.10. overtime salaries for employees to temporarily fill vacancy	a. direct costs
____ 17.11. equipment damage	b. indirect costs
____ 17.12. orientation	
____ 17.13. lowered personnel morale	
____ 17.14. position advertising costs	

APPLICATION, ANALYSIS, AND/OR SYNTHESIS

Multiple Choice

17.15. Which of the following will be most useful for Nurse Manager Upncomer to use when analyzing the unit turnover rate?
 a. compare the unit turnover rate with turnover rates of other units in her facility
 b. compare the unit turnover rate with the turnover rate at a similar unit in another facility
 c. compare the unit turnover rate with national turnover rates for like facilities
 d. compare the numbers of voluntary and involuntary resignations for the facility

17.16. Which of the following represents data Nurse Manager Upncomer will use when computing the unit annual turnover rate?
 a. number of unit full-time equivalent positions
 b. number of employees retained
 c. average number of unit employees
 d. all of above

17.17. Nurse Manager Upncomer notices that 60% of the new graduates from the area BSN school quit after 9 to 12 months of employment. Which action(s) would be appropriate?
 a. clear representation of expected job activities during recruitment
 b. compare staffing patterns with schooling practices
 c. share sample work schedules during interview process
 d. all of above

17.18. Nurse Manager Upncomer examines staffing practices for the purpose of lowering a high turnover rate. Which of the following would most likely promote staff retention?
 a. nursing care delivery mode that pairs experienced nurse with a new nurse
 b. employee goal setting
 c. career ladder programs built upon employee performance - professional growth
 d. all of above

17.19. Nurse Manager Upncomer decides that exit interviews should be conducted with staff who resign during the next six months. To promote useful exit interview data, Ms. Upncomer will do which of the following?
   a. post a notice stating she will interview all employees at the time of their resignation
   b. appoint a unit staff ad hoc committee of three to conduct exit interviews
   c. request that the personnel department conduct exit interviews for the next six months
   d. all of above

17.20. Which of the following represent recruitment activities which promote staff retention?
   a. recruitment material is written to include negative and positive aspects of the position
   b. tour unit to observe personnel performing typical tasks
   c. redesign orientation program to match individual employee needs
   d. all of above

17.21. Which of the following managerial practices will promote staff retention?
   a. the new employee is allowed flexibility of scheduling hours which has not been practiced
   b. new graduate employees are assigned to exciting positions in intensive care and the trauma center
   c. use clear performance standards for job evaluations
   d. all of above

Matching: Match the correct term to the event by placing the appropriate letter in the space provided. You may use a term more than once.

Event

____ 17.22. The percentage of employed nurses separated from their jobs during the quarter was

____ 17.23. Husband accepts position in a different city, so nurse resigns.

____ 17.24. The staff nurse complained that the relief nurse manager expected her to do different assignments than the regular nurse manager.

____ 17.25. Nurse quits to care for baby.

____ 17.26. The written job description included different performance standards than those practiced.

____ 17.27. The patient census was so low that the unit was closed and the nurse manager was laid off.

____ 17.28. The newly graduated nurse expected to be able to sit down and talk with patients, but found she did not have time.

Term

a. involuntary turnover

b. role ambiguity

c. role conflict

d. turnover

e. voluntary turnover

ANSWERS	TEXT REFERENCE
17.01. T	p. 292
17.02. F	p. 293
17.03. T	p. 295
17.04. T	p. 295
17.05. T	p. 299
17.06. F	p. 300
17.07. F	p. 300
17.08. d	p. 293
17.09. b	p. 294
17.10. b	p. 293
17.11. b	p. 293
17.12. a	p. 293
17.13. b	p. 293
17.14. a	p. 293
17.15. a	p. 292, 293
17.16. c	p. 293
17.17. d	p. 295
17.18. d	p. 294, 295
17.19. c	p. 297
17.20. d	p. 298
17.21. c	p. 295, 299
17.22. a	p. 293
17.23. a	p. 2293
17.24. c	p. 295
17.25. e	p. 293
17.26. b	p. 295
17.27. a	p. 293
17.28. c	p. 295

CHAPTER

18

Staff Development

Rapid societal, technological, and medical advancements compel nursing administration to place a high value upon staff development. The contents of this chapter provide both an overview and specific considerations applicable to staff development activities. Figure 18.1 (at the end of this Manual) will help students recognize the considerable costs involved in educational programming.

KEY TERMS

adaptive learning
andragogy
fixed costs
"flow"
learning module
role modeling
role playing
sunk costs
T-groups
variable costs

OUTLINE

I. Overview
  A. Description of staff development
  B. Need for staff development
    1. Societal change
    2. Scientific change
    3. Ancillary nursing personnel
    4. Collective bargaining
    5. Promote productivity
    6. New practice roles
    7. Staff vitality
    8. Accreditation and regulatory requirements
II. Types of staff development
  A. Definition of staff development
  B. Goals of staff development
  C. Descriptions of activities
    1. Induction training
    2. Orientation
    3. Inservice education
    4. Continuing education
  D. Internal credentialing system
III. Staff development concepts
  A. Terms illustrated
    1. Competence
    2. Interests
    3. Need
    4. Learning
      a. Informal learning
      b. Technical learning
  B. Adult learners
    1. Types of adult learning

   2. Malcolm Knowles
  C. Educational concepts and principles
   1. Ultimate responsibility rests with employee
   2. Learning combines experience and conceptualization
   3. Learning is an internal, personal, and emotional process
   4. Learning is a behavioral change
   5. Adults are autonomous learners
   6. Adult learning is promoted through application
   7. Positive immediate rewards promote repetition
   8. Aspects of learning are organized into an integrated whole
   9. Transfer of learning is maximized through use of realistic simulation
   10. Transfer of learning is maximized when behavioral changes are rewarded
   11. Learning is active rather than passive
   12. Adults are self-directed learners building on life experiences
    a. Life experiences may inhibit or promote learning
   13. Adult learners are a heterogeneous group

IV. Stages of adult occupational development
  A. Stages ascribed to age ranges
  B. Motivation stimuli
   1. Economic
   2. Self-actualization
   3. Extrinsic-intrinsic factors
   4. "Flow"

V. Organizing staff development resources
  A. Place in agency
  B. Use of "pool" specialists
  C. Liaison with area colleges

VI. Quality control of continuing education courses
  A. American Nurses' Association
   1. Accredits CEUs
  B. National League for Nursing
   1. Accredits academic credit courses

VII. Staff development advisory committee
  A. Purpose
  B. Composition
  C. Function
  D. Planning
  E. Accountability

VIII. Cost of staff development activities
  A. Cost:benefit analysis
  B. Types of costs
   1. Sunk costs
   2. Fixed costs
   3. Variable costs
   4. Unit costs
  D. Use of external consultant
  E. Cost accounting

IX. Guidelines for staff development programs
  A. CEU credit
  B. Program outline
  C. Outcome evaluation
  D. Criteria for instructors
  E. Roles of committee members
  F. Agency members as teachers

X. The staff development instructor
  A. Needed strengths
  B. Facilitator of discovery learning
  C. Coaching role
  D. Role modeling
   1. Direct
   2. Indirect

XI. Organization of staff development personnel
  A. Basic level teachers
  B. Advanced level teachers

XII. Preferred topics for staff development programs
  A. Poll employees
  B. Identified skill needs
  C. Problem alleviation

XIII. Planning for staff development programs
  A. Course objectives
  B. Example given

XIV. Levels of learning
  A. Memorization and simple motor response
  B. Adaptive
  C. Isolation and integration of select learning
  D. Integration of values and learning needs

XV. Teaching methods and aids
  A. Teaching methods defined
   1. Lecture
   2. Discussion
   3. Media
   4. Learning module
   5. Role playing and simulation
   6. Role modeling
   7. Management games

- B. Audiovisual equipment for staff development
  - 1. Use of multiple senses
  - 2. Principles for self-study
    - a. Learner motivation
    - b. Material organization
    - c. Repetition
    - d. Prompt feedback
  - 3. List of needed hardware
- C. Preparation of audiovisual materials
  - 1. Use of media specialist
  - 2. Module content

XVI. Orientation
- A. Purpose
- B. Goals
- C. Relationship to job description
- D. Manual

XVII. Nurse internship
- A. Purposes
- B. Description
- C. Examples

XVIII. Career mobility program
- A. Purposes
  - 1. Increase morale
  - 2. Decrease turnover
- B. Degree mobility
- C. Examples

XIX. Inservice education
- A. Purpose
- B. JCAHO requirements
- C. Merging centralized and decentralized educational practices
- D. Guidelines

XX. Management development
- A. Need for democratic leadership
- B. Need for different perspective
- C. Systems approach
  - 1. Delineation of each management level
  - 2. Effectiveness evaluations
  - 3. Problem/needs identification
  - 4. Educational programming
    - a. Use of immediate supervisor
    - b. Topics
    - c. Group dynamics
    - d. Scope
    - e. Academic courses
- D. Coaching
  - 1. Base on trust
  - 2. Knowledge of learner's strengths and weaknesses
  - 3. Content versus process analysis
  - 4. Planning technique
- E. Decision making
- F. Communication
- G. Use of job rotation
- H. Management games
- I. Identification of manager learning needs
  - 1. Promotion patterns
  - 2. Development needs by management levels
- J. Program examples
- K. Mentoring
  - 1. Role of mentor
  - 2. Benefits of mentoring

XXI. Organization development
- A. Defined
- B. Activities listed
- C. Critical elements
  - 1. Accurate diagnosis
  - 2. Appropriate interventions

XXII. Teambuilding
- A. Use of workshops
- B. Grid approach
  - 1. Love-trust
  - 2. Power-coercive
  - 3. Insight-consensus
- C. Use of group dynamics
  - 1. Feedback
  - 2. Disclosure
  - 3. T-groups

XXIII. Summary

DISCUSSION IDEA: Costing educational programs

Nurses who have not had an opportunity to work with educational programming will profit by considering the many costs involved. Figure 18.1 may be copied as an overhead or for distribution to students to illustrate how educational program costs may be estimated, and recorded; and how estimated and actual costs can be compared.

DISCUSSION IDEA: Employee Participation in Educational Activities

Objective 1: Explain how induction learning and inservice education stimulate staff members to develop new knowledge and skills.

Ask students to imagine that they are graduated and hired to a position that is new to them. Ask students to write down two topics for induction, and two inservice topics which they feel would aid them in the position.

Ask for several student volunteers to share the job title and topics they have identified.

Ask students how they would feel if they were given the same opportunity of identifying topics in a real situation.

GROUP ACTIVITIES: Continuing Education for Nurse Managers: A Readiness Program

A readiness program is designed for the purpose of growing staff in anticipation of need. Staff have the opportunity of choosing areas in which they are interested in growing and thus staff morale is increased. The agency has the benefit of increased staff expertise and knowledge both prior to and at time of change in position. A pool of staff prepared in areas of potential need is a strong benefit of readiness programming.

Situation: Podville Hospital's Over 70s unit
Position: Nurse Unit Manager

Podville Hospital offers "readiness" educational programming. The content of the readiness programs is based upon entry level knowledge and skills needed for specific positions. A Nurse Unit Manager Readiness program is the educational focus with which these activities are concerned.

Resource: Text pages 322-326.

Activity : Preservice Education Readiness Program for Nurse Unit Managers

1. List 6-8 preservice education content for a nurse manager readiness program for the position of Nurse Unit Manager

2. List demonstrated outcomes for each of the content items identified above.

3. State three educational methods which could be used in implementing a preservice education readiness program for Nurse Unit Managers.

4. Identify three adult education principles which may be incorporated.

GROUP ACTIVITY: Inservice Education for Nurse Unit Managers

Objective 2 is applied in the activity.

Objective 2: Enumerate three adult learning principles to be followed in providing in-service instruction to nurses.

1. Assume that Podville Nurse Unit Managers have each completed the Preservice Education Management Readiness program, and are now on the job.

   Identify five topics which would be appropriate for Nurse Unit Manager inservice education?

   What might be three educational methods particularly applicable for this population?

2. An experienced Nurse Unit Manager was hired from outside the facility, and has not participated in the Management Readiness program.

   In designing an orientation program for the new manager what are three areas that should be included? (Induction to facility, specific to assigned unit, tailored management skills and information.)

ASSIGNMENTS

Chapter objectives 3 and 4 may each be used as assignments.

Objective 3: Identify educational programs offered by local colleges, community agencies, and professional organizations that could be used as staff development activities for nurses in your agency.

Assignment

1. Have students list nursing staff development activities offered in the community.
2. What types of institutions offer staff development activities for nurses?
3. Which activities would be appropriate for nurse managers?

Objective 4: Review the course outline for a nursing inservice program, and evaluate whether objectives, content, teachers, methods, materials, and time allotment are appropriate for the program's purpose.

Provide students with a copy of a course outline for a nursing inservice program, preferably one which is suitable for nurse managers. Designate a nurse management position with which they are familiar.

Assignment

Critique the inservice program in relation to the nurse manager in the designated position.

Are course objectives useful and applicable to position?

Is course content useful and applicable to position?

Is faculty appropriate for the content?

Are teaching methods used appropriate for adult learners?

Is time allotment adequate to meet stated objectives?

TEST QUESTIONS

KNOWLEDGE AND COMPREHENSION

True : False

T F 18.01. Andragogy is the art and science of teaching.

T F 18.02. The ultimate responsibility for professional development rests with the employee.

T F 18.03. Adults learn best when lesson content can be applied immediately.

T F 18.04. Adults with less than 12 years of schooling usually return to school to satisfy self-actualizing needs.

T F 18.05. The role of staff development teacher is information giver and expert.

T F 18.06. Course objectives should state exact expected participant behaviors.

T F 18.07. A desired outcome of a career mobility program is to decrease nurse turnover.

T F 18.08. Enhancing management skills of the highest level of administration will produce the greatest improvement in patient services.

T F 18.09. The first step in a management development program is agreement as to proper level of authority, responsibility and accountability at every level.

Multiple Choice

18.10. Need for staff development activities arises because of
a. rapid societal changes
b. advances in health science
c. need to increase productivity
d. accreditation requirements
e. all of above

18.11. The individual who finds internal pleasure and becomes "lost" in the excitement and discovery of learning is said to experience:
a. appropriate adult education
b. technical learning
c. "flow"
d. all of above

18.12. Which of the following organizations accredits educational programs that grant continuing education units to nurses?
a. American Nurses' Association
b. National League for Nursing
c. all State Boards of Nursing
d. National Nursing Research Association

18.13. The role of the staff development advisory committee includes:
a. establish guidelines for educational use
b. evaluate educational program outcomes
c. establish criteria for selecting instructors
d. all of above

18.14. Which of the following behaviors will contribute(s) to being a successful staff development teacher? The teacher:
a. focuses on the trainee's abilities and potential.
b. demonstrates how to extract information from unit resources.
c. uses patient care problems from trainees' units.
d. all of above

18.15. Which type of learning is demonstrated by the nurse who memorizes common dosages of the most frequently ordered medications?
a. first level
b. adaptive learning
c. integrated learning
d. values integration

18.16. Which type of learning is demonstrated when the information at the workshop is applied a bit differently on the unit?
a. first level
b. adaptive learning
c. integrated learning
d. values integration

18.17. Which type of learning is demonstrated when the janitor performed emergency CPR on a visitor in the lobby following an all employee CPR program?
a. first level
b. adaptive learning
c. integrated learning
d. values integration

18.18. A mentor serves as a:
a. sponsor
b. role model
c. advocate
d. all of above

18.19. The purpose(s) of a nurse internship include(s):
a. enhancement of recruitment
b. facilitate transition of new graduate from student to nurse role
c. decrease head nurse time spent on basic skill training
d. all of above

Matching: Match the teaching/learning method to characteristics by placing the appropriate letter in the space provided.

Characteristics	Teaching/Learning Method
___ 18.20. The student is an admitted novice, the teacher is a recognized expert.	a. case studies
___ 18.21. Contain materials and exercises for a narrow content area.	b. games
___ 18.22. Allows student to confront a series of complex problems, and make decision without risk.	c. learning module
___ 18.23. Teaches problem-solving techniques.	d. role modeling
___ 18.24. The learner can experiment with problem solving approaches.	e. simulation

APPLICATION, ANALYSIS, AND/OR SYNTHESIS

Matching: Match the type of staff development programming to the program content by placing the correct letter in the space provided.

Program Content

____ 18.25. High risk procedure skill verification program for emergency room nurses

____ 18.26. Facility philosophy, policies

____ 18.27. How to prepare a unit budget

____ 18.28. How to enter a nursing care plan into an established computer system

____ 18.29. New "code" procedures for all nurses

Type of Staff Development Program

a. continuing education

b. induction

c. inservice education

d. orientation

Matching: Match the term which best relates to the practice example by placing the appropriate letter in the space provided. Use each answer only once.

Practice Example

___ 18.30. The new unit manager who varies management style to match employee needs is demonstrating _?_.

___ 18.31. The staff nurse who twice asked the unit manager when the inservice on the new computer program is scheduled is demonstrating _?_.

___ 18.32. The new nurse manager does not know how to run the new computer program. She is demonstrating _?_.

___ 18.33. The performance of the LPN paired with Nurse Icandoit improved markedly in the last performance evaluation period. The LPN is most likely demonstrating _?_.

___ 18.34. After the inservice, the I & O records done by the nursing assistants were more accurate. The nursing assistants are demonstrating _?_.

Term

a. competence

b. informal learning

c. interest

d. need

e. technical learning

Matching: Match the term to the appropriate example by placing the letter in the space provided. Terms may be used more than once.

Examples

____ 18.35. Honorarium paid to guest lecturer.

____ 18.36. Price of purchased large screen TV.

____ 18.37. Refreshments at conference.

____ 18.38. Encumbered money for a new video camera.

____ 18.39. Handouts for workshop.

____ 18.40. Amount spent per participating employee.

Terms

a. fixed costs

b. sunk costs

c. unit costs

d. variable costs

Multiple Choice

18.41. Which of the following best illustrates the achievement of *the primary* goal of staff development?
- a. staff nurse follows new procedure correctly
- b. all departmental heads attended the management inservice
- c. staff nurse is observed using the library to learn more about topic
- d. the unit manager said she would start the new process next month

18.42. Which of the following are likely to be positively received by the adult nurse learner?
- a. the central education office provides a list of educational needs to the nurses
- b. administration will present certificates of recognition for educational participation every two years
- c. the nurse identifies own strengths and needs
- d. all of above

18.43. Which of the following educational activities is most likely to produce improvement in identifying abnormal ECGs in the cardiac intensive care unit?
- a. A CEU offering is given at the local community college showing ECG slides and discussing what the slides are showing.
- b. Weekly walking round "case studies" in the unit targeting persons with abnormal ECGs.
- c. The unit manager orders two copies of a highly recommended book on ECG interpretation.
- d. The agency inservice educator offers a program on ECG interpretation.

18.44. Which of the following topics would most likely be received positively by staff?
- a. The topics were identified by polling staff.
- b. The unit managers identified topics contributing to poor productivity.
- c. The topics were identified through quality control activities.
- d. Administration identified topics pertaining to cost:benefit problems.

ANSWERS	TEXT REFERENCE
18.01. F	p. 308
18.02. T	p. 308
18.03. T	p. 309
18.04. F	p. 310
18.05. F	p. 315
18.06. T	p. 317
18.07. T	p. 320
18.08. F	p. 322
18.09. T	p. 322
18.10. e	p. 305, 306
18.11. c	p. 310
18.12. a	p. 312
18.13. d	p. 312
18.14. e	p. 314, 315
18.15. a	p. 317
18.16. b	p. 318
18.17. b	p. 318
18.18. d	p. 326
18.19. d	p. 319, 320
18.20. d	p. 318
18.21. c	p. 318
18.22. b	p. 318
18.23. a	p. 317, 318
18.24. e	p. 318
18.25. c	p. 307, 321
18.26. b	p. 306, 307
18.27. a	p. 307
18.28. d	p. 307, 319
18.29. c	p. 307, 321
18.30. a	p. 308
18.31. c	p. 308
18.32. d	p. 308
18.33. b	p. 308
18.34. e	p. 308
18.35. a	p. 313
18.36. b	p. 313
18.37. d	p. 313
18.38. b	p. 313
18.39. d	p. 313
18.40. c	p. 313
18.41. c	p. 308
18.42. c	p. 308-310
18.43. b	p. 309
18.44. a	p. 316

CHAPTER

19

Leading

A leader is not necessarily a manager, and a manager is not necessarily a leader. However, a good manager is able to lead subordinates. This chapter contains different approaches to leadership and helpful explication of leadership roles and methods in relation to positions in the nursing hierarchy.

KEY TERMS

autocratic style
burnout
contingency
democratic style
laissez faire style
leader
leadership style
manager
reinforcement
situation theory
supervision
transactional leader
transformational leader

OUTLINE

I. Introduction
 A. Management process reviewed
 B. "To lead" defined
 C. Characteristics of an effective leader

II. Leadership activities
 A. Directing
 B. Supervising
 C. Coordinating

III. Leadership roles
 A. Transformational leader
 B. Transactional leader
 C. Management hierarchy
  1. Executive
  2. Top Level: Administrator
  3. Middle level: Supervisor, divisional director
  4. First level: Head Nurse, patient care manager
 D. Expectations of managers
 E. Biculturalism of first-level managers
 F. Leadership and change

IV. Relation of leadership to other management functions
 A. Management process preceding project

   B. Sequential management process steps responsibility of different management levels
   C. Management process steps conducted concurrently

V. The first-level manager
   A. Responsibilities
      1. Ensure safe and effective care delivery
      2. Protect employee welfare
   B. Leadership behavior
   C. Role in institutional "status quo"
      1. Adherence to institutional systems
      2. Reordering priorities to meet needs
      3. Creative problem solving
      4. Decision making
      5. Use data

VI. Leadership styles
   A. Style defined
   B. Style types
      1. Autocratic
      2. Democratic
      3. Participative
      4. Laissez faire
   C. Impact of leadership style
   D. "Best" leadership style factors

VII. Contingency or situation theory of leadership
   A. Overview
   B. Goal priority
   C. Adapting leadership style to situation
   D. Success dependent upon style match
      1. Relationship oriented
      2. Task oriented

VIII. Direction
   A. Types
   B. Style and use
   C. Orders
      1. Definition
      2. Types
         a. Written
         b. Oral
      3. Style
      4. Frequency
      5. Content
      6. Sender-receiver distance
      7. Depersonalizing orders
      8. Avoidance of order giving

IX. Supervision (Overseeing)
   A. Overview
      1. Definition
      2. Purpose
      3. Intensity
      4. Span
      5. Appraisal criteria
   B. Supervision as coaching
      1. Goals
      2. Techniques
   C. Supervision as control
   D. Supervisory techniques
      1. Observation
      2. Task assistance
      3. Correction
      4. Spot-checking
      5. Questioning
   E. Correcting performance
      1. Individualize methods
      2. Use of case study
      3. Use of institutional goals
      4. Use of job descriptions
      5. Confrontation
      6. Morale issue
      7. Scheduling of supervision
   F. Chemical dependency
      1. Occurrence
      2. Stages
      3. Signs
      4. Confrontation
      5. Return-to-work contract
      6. Recovery stages
         a. Premotivation
         b. Breakthrough
         c. Early recovery
         d. Extended recovery
      7. Interview focus

X. Protecting personnel from hazards
   A. Physical trauma
      1. Types
         a. Assistive equipment
         b. Assault evaluation
      2. Occurrence
      3. Preventive measures
   B. Toxicological injury
      1. Examples of toxic substances
      2. Types of injuries
   C. Infection
      1. Examples of infections
      2. Preventive measures
   D. AIDS
      1. Universal blood and body fluid precautions
      2. Limitations
   E. Stress
      1. Contributing factors
      2. Stress behaviors

3. Manager responses

F. Stress caused by AIDS
   1. Nurse depression
   2. AIDS stigma
   3. Fear of contacting AIDS
   4. Interventions
   5. Agency provided health services for nurses

XI. Coordination
   A. Definition
   B. Diversity of employee styles
      1. Style examples
         a. Self-reliant
         b. Enthusiastic
         c. Loyal
         d. Factual
      2. Team building
      3. Integration
   C. Communication
      1. Memoranda
      2. Posters
      3. Position paper
      4. Group dynamics
      5. Meetings

XII. Motivating
   A. Overview
   B. Promoting motivation
   C. Need theories
      1. Maslow's hierarchy of needs
      2. Herzberg's two factor theory
      3. McClelland's theory
         a. Achievement needs
         b. Affiliation needs
         c. Power needs
   C. Operant theory
      1. Skinner
      2. Reinforcement
   D. Expectancy theory
      1. Vroom
      2. Porter and Lawler
      3. House
   E. Equity theory (Adams)
   F. Competence theory (White)
   G. Job satisfaction and motivation
      1. Research findings
      2. Dimensions of job satisfaction
      3. Dissatisfiers
      4. Job related stress
         a. Selye's three phases
         b. Frain and Valigna's four categories
         c. "Burnout"
            (1). Symptoms
            (2). Occurrence
            (3). Relation to job dissatisfaction
         d. Sources
   H. Preventing and relieving stress and burnout
      1. Educational approaches
      2. Support groups
      3. Support programs
      4. Remedy through job design, organizational structure
   I. Increasing motivation through job redesign
      1. Job rotation
      2. Job enlargement
      3. Job enrichment
         a. Research findings
         b. Guidelines
   J. Clinical ladder systems
      1. Description
      2. Limited research

XIII. Summary

DISCUSSION IDEA: Motivation

Objective 1 may be used as a discussion topic.

Objective 1: Contrast the motivations of a leader with those of a manager.

DISCUSSION IDEAS: Leadership

Chapter objective 2: Contrast the methods used by a leader and manager to secure subordinates' compliance with agency goals.

1. What methods might a nurse manager use that a non-management nurse leader cannot use?

   Chapter objective 3: Explain the double bind in which managers are caught because of their position in the organizational hierarchy.

2. Imagine yourself as a nurse unit manager during labor contract negotiations. What would be the staff nurses' expectancies of you during negotiations?

   What would be administration's expectancies of you during negotiations?

ASSIGNMENT: Leadership Style

Leadership styles should match employee needs. One method of considering leadership styles is to consider the amount of focus and support the manager displays in task matters or in relationships. A manager may place high or low emphasis on tasks and on relationships. Discuss the preferred style of management task and relationship behaviors for each of the following situations. Give rational for your answers.

1. Situation: Unit manager orienting a newly certificated nursing assistant to the unit.

Questions

a. What would most likely happen if the unit manager practiced a low task and low relationship style?

   (Response: The nursing assistant's needs will not be met. The nursing assistant will not be satisfied with employment situation, and will look for needs to be satisfied elsewhere.)

b. How might the nursing assistant respond to a high task, low relationship style?

   (Response: The nursing assistant likely needs both high task and high relationship needs. The nursing assistant will look elsewhere for high relationship needs which will be found in an astute unit leader. This may become a future problem to the manager.)

c. Which style would be best?

(Response: High task and high relationship until employee feels secure.)

2. Situation: Unit manager is assigned to work with consultant who is conducting time studies.

Questions

a. Would the consultant be helped by a high task high relationship style on the part of the unit manager?

(Response: No. A high relationship style would likely impede the consultant's work.)

b. Which unit manager leadership style would best facilitate the consultant's work?

(Response: low task, low relationship.)

3. Situation: Experienced staff nurse transfers to the unit.

Questions

a. What style would best be practiced by the unit manager?

(Preferred style would be variable. The unit manager would be wise to ask the nurse what she needs. The first day or two the unit manager will need to be sensitive to both high task and high relationship needs. The unit manager will likely need to be sensitive to quickly lowering task foci, while providing a bit longer for relationship needs on the unit. The unit manager needs to feel comfortable both stepping into and out of high task and relationship interactions.)

TEST QUESTIONS

KNOWLEDGE AND COMPREHENSION

True : False

T F 19.01. Leadership is influencing the behavior of others through social relationships.

T F 19.02. A nurse manager's non-programmed decisions should be data based, not opinion based.

T F 19.03. A leader's power to command the behavior of others derives from his/her knowledge base.

T F 19.04. The most effective supervision is based on the philosophy and techniques of sports coaching.

T F 19.05. Performance observation is the preferred way to supervise a professional nurse.

T F 19.06. Confrontation is required when a subordinate continues to perform inadequately even though counseled and instructed.

T F 19.07. The rate of chemical dependency in nurses is approximately one in ten.

T F 19.08. Nurse anesthetists are subject to perceptual, cognitive and motor impairment with repeated exposure to anesthetic gases.

T F 19.09. In coordinating the efforts of the many health care specialist the nurse manager should use clearly stated orders.

T F 19.10. According to McClelland's motivation research a nurse manager can increase the achievement need of unproductive staff members through appropriate staff development programs.

T F 19.11. There is evidence that job stress and job dissatisfaction decrease nurses' work motivation.

T F 19.12. A clinical ladder system rewards nurses by moving them into management positions.

Matching: Match the role of the nursing leader or nursing manager to the action or responsibility by placing the relevant letter in the space provided. Use an answer only once.

Action/Responsibility	Role
____ 19.13. synthesizes efforts of others	a. nursing executive
____ 19.14. a middle manager	b. nursing leader
____ 19.15. top-level manager	c. nursing manager
____ 19.16. first-line manager	d. nursing supervisor
____ 19.17. rewards worker's efforts toward goal achievement	e. head nurse

Multiple Choice

19.18. The three major leadership behaviors are:
a. order giving, information gathering, evaluation
b. planning, delegating, distributing resources
c. directing, supervising, coordinating
d. teaching, disciplining, goal setting

19.19. The text refers to the fact that nurse managers find themselves in a "double-bind" because of organizational hierarchy. Which of the following best represents this biculturalism?
a. superior or administrative, and subordinate or labor expectancies are different
b. the manager is both a leader and a disciplinarian
c. the manager is always to work through others
d. personal and institutional goals are mismatched

19.20. To *lead* a clinical unit effectively, a manager must be:
a. an accepted member of the group
b. perceived as superior to other members
c. have ideals and professional interests that resemble those of the subordinates
d. all of above

19.19. Managers can increase their power by:
a. delegating decisions to subordinates
b. socializing freely with subordinates
c. requiring all information be channeled through them
d. all of above

19.22. The theory that views successful management as a proper match between the manager's leadership style and the amount of manager control is:
a. democratic leadership
b. Feidler's contingency theory
c. House's path-goal theory
d. McClelland's theory

19.23. Which leadership style is best in an emergency?
a. autocratic
b. democratic
c. participative
d. laissez faire

19.24. Which of the following will increase the clarity of a written message?
a. specify desired task in behavioral terms
b. designate time limits
c. provide standards for task
d. a and c only
e. all of above

19.25. Leadership research shows that a leader's behavior is perceived positively by subordinates if it:
a. meets immediate needs of subordinates
b. facilitates subordinates in meeting institutional goals
c. increases likelihood of subordinates reaching long-term goals
d. a and c only
e. all of above

19.26. Typical signs of chemical dependency include:
a. frequent tardiness
b. rapid mood swings
c. frequent errors and accidents
d. a and c only
e. all of above

APPLICATION, ANALYSIS, AND/OR SYNTHESIS

Matching: Match the leadership style to the behavioral example by placing the relevant letter in the space provided.

	Behavioral example	Leadership Style
____	19.27. The nurse administrator leaves direction, decision making, and coordination up to the nurse unit managers.	a. autocratic
		b. democratic
____	19.28. The nurse administrator writes and distributes unit goals to the unit managers.	c. laissez faire
		d. participative
____	19.29. The nurse administrator presents her analyses of the problem and possible solutions, but leaves the final decision to unit managers.	

Matching: Match the theory or theorist which the motivating action is practicing by placing the appropriate letter in the space provided. An answer may be used more than once.

Motivating Action

____ 19.30. Nurse manager compliments staff on a job well done.

____ 19.31. The staff are dissatisfied with working conditions and thus are not motivated to work at their best.

____ 19.32. The nurse takes a break to put her feet up before caring for a difficult patient is demonstrating ?

____ 19.33. The nurse who acquires a clinical masters degree before applying for a position in that clinical area is demonstrating a high achievement need according to ?

____ 19.34. Nurse Quzee anticipates a merit raise for her conscientious work during the last evaluation period.

____ 19.35. The nurse manager submits a policy recommendation to abolish raises for seniority and to link raises to performance.

____ 19.36. The nurse administrator who re designed the unit manager position to include greater autonomy and authority is practicing ?

Theory/Theorist

a. Adam's equity

b. Herzberg's factor

c. Maslow's needs hierarchy

d. McClelland

e. Operant

Multiple Choice

19.37. Which of the following orders will minimize interpersonal friction?
a. "Francis, will you take the specimen to the lab for me right now?"
b. "Can I count on you to work the holiday?"
c. "Do me a favor and answer Mr. Green's light."
d. "OR called for Mr. Morris. Please take him to OR right away."

19.38. Which of the following would increase the supervisor's effectiveness?
a. "Why do you do it that way?"
b. "Hazel did it an easier way, let me show you."
c. "That's not a good way to do it."
d. "Where did you learn that?"

19.39. Which of the following illustrate the purpose of supervision?
a. The manager reviews the service units provided to personnel on duty ratio.
b. The manager asks the quality review committee to review the critical indicator for urinary tract infections for the last two weeks and consecutively.
c. The manager compares budgeted monies and monies spent on disposable supplies.
d. a and c only
e. all of above

19.40. Which of the following may be symptoms of psychosocial distress?
a. Nurse Matilda volunteers for extra work.
b. Nurse Henry, a star bowler, has been absent from the unit bowling league.
c. The staff nurse has frequent mood changes.
d. a and c only
e. all of above

19.41. Which of the following would alert the nurse manager to possible employee burnout?
a. Nurse Ohmy is unable to complete her assignments in a timely manner.
b. Nurse Metoo submits a request to attend an ICU workshop in hopes of transferring to ICU.
c. The nurse was overhears to disdainfully say of the patient, "She just is looking for something to complain about. She's OK."
d. a and c only
e. all of above

ANSWERS	TEXT REFERENCE
19.01. T	p. 333
19.02. T	p. 337
19.03. F	p. 340
19.04. T	p. 344
19.05. F	p. 345
19.06. T	p. 346
19.07. F	p. 345
19.08. T	p. 349
19.09. F	p. 353
19.10. T	p. 355
19.11. T	p. 358
19.12. F	p. 361
19.13. b	p. 333
19.14. d	p. 334
19.15. a	p. 334
19.16. e	p. 334
19.17. c	p. 334
19.18. c	p. 334
19.19. a	p. 335, 336
19.20. d	p. 339
19.19. c	p. 340
19.22. b	p. 340
19.23. a	p. 340
19.24. e	p. 341
19.25. d	p. 344
19.26. e	p. 347
19.27. c	p. 338
19.28. a	p. 338
19.29. d	p. 338
19.30. e	p. 356
19.31. b	p. 354
19.32. c	p. 354
19.33. d	p. 355
19.34. f	p. 356
19.35. a	p. 356
19.36. b	p. 360
19.37. d	p. 342
19.38. b	p. 344
19.39. e	p. 343, 344
19.40. e	p. 350
19.41. d	p. 358

CHAPTER

20

Nursing Ethics

Limited resources, both dollar and personnel, create many ethical dilemmas for the nurse manager. Changing heath care technologies, changing societal norms and expectancies, and an aging population create many unresolved ethical conflicts for the caregiver. Chapter 20 offers an overview of ethical principles and applications in health care settings. The content provides a structure within which ethical issues may be deliberated and a basis for better informed decision making.

KEY TERMS

attitude
autonomy
belief
beneficence
coercion
concept
deception
deontological ethics
duty
ethicist
ethics
fidelity
fiduciary
goodness
lying
justice
need
nonmaleficence
principle
right
teleological ethic
theory
utility
value
veracity

OUTLINE

I. Overview
  A. Definitions
  B. Beliefs and values
    1. Development of
    2. Incongruence of

II. Universal moral principles
  A. Autonomy
    1. Definition of
    2. Respect for
    3. Types of

a. Freedom of action
b. Freedom of choice
c. Effective deliberation
4. Deterrents to
a. Coercion
b. Incomplete or misinformation
c. Limiting care options
5. Informed consent
B. Freedom
1. Description
2. Choice
3. Viewpoints
a. Hard determinists
b. Libertarians
4. Practice examples
C. Veracity
1. Responsibility of caregivers
2. Impact of truthtelling
3. Difficulties in truthtelling
a. Negative diagnosis
b. Time limitations
c. Denial of patient desires
d. Lying and deception
D. Justice
1. Definition of justice
2. Questions of justice
3. Principles of fair distribution
4. Compensatory justice
5. Retributive justice
E. Nonmaleficence
1. Definition
2. Sanctity of human life
F. Beneficence
1. Definition
2. Principles
a. Provision of enhancing benefits
b. Balancing of benefit and harms
3. Relationship to nonmaleficence
G. Right
1. Definition
2. Conventional rights
3. Moral rights

III. Approaches to ethical decision making
A. Descriptive ethics
B. Normative ethics
1. Defined
2. Divisions
a. Norms of value
b. Norms of obligation
3. Schools
a. Deontological ethics
b. Teleological ethics
C. Assessment criteria for competing theories
1. Internal consistency
2. Degree of simplicity
3. Extent of agreement
4. Extent of guidance
D. Utilitarianism
1. Defined
2. Application
a. Act utilitarianism
b. Rule utilitarianism
3. Universalizability
E. Kant's categorical imperative
1. Fundamental principle
2. Four additional principles
3. Applications

IV. Ethical codes
A. Nurenberg Code
1. History
2. Criteria for human research
B. Declaration of Helsinki
1. Tenets for biomedical research
2. Institutional application
C. Codes for Medical Professionals
1. Hippocratic oath
2. American Medical Association
3. American College of Healthcare Executives
4. American Nurses' Association Code of Ethics for Nurses

V. Ethical dilemmas for nurses
A. Examples of dilemmas
B. Need for ethical decision making
C. Rationing nursing care
1. Methods for rationing
a. Market rationing
b. Explicit rationing
c. Implicit rationing
2. Examples of theory application to care rationing
D. Quality of life concept to ration care
1. Defining characteristics
2. Measuring quality of life
a. Research methods and findings
b. Quality adjusted life years
(1). Description
(2). Impact
(3). Relationship to ethical principles

E. Treatment decisions for incurable terminally ill
   1. Definitions of death
   2. Prestated wishes of terminally ill
   3. "Whole brain dead" proposal
   4. Life sustaining measures
      a. Ordinary
      b. Extraordinary
   5. DNR orders
   6. Suicide
   7. Euthanasia
      a. Passive
      b. Active
      c. Aid-in-dying Act
F. Obtaining informed consent for treatment and research
   1. Ethical principles
      a. Autonomy
      b. Nonmaleficence
   2. Arguments regarding children
G. Confidentiality and privacy concerns
   1. Right to privacy
   2. Patient's chart

VI. Summary

CLASS DISCUSSION: Ethical Dilemmas

Choose one of the situations presented in the Memo Capsule on page 383 of the text.

Questions

1. Which ethical principles apply to the situation?
2. How would you respond?

   Give rationale, including ethical principles, which you used in making decision.

ASSIGNMENT: Ethical Dilemmas

After completing the above discussion as an example, ask students to choose one of the remaining situations presented in the Memo Capsule on page 383 of the text.

The assignment relates to chapter objective 1: Describe two ethical dilemmas that nurses encounter concerning treatment decisions for patients.

Assignment: In one typewritten page:

1. Which ethical principles apply to the situation?
2. How would you respond?

   Give rationale including ethical principles which you used in making decision.

GROUP DISCUSSION: Ethical Principles and Management Decisions

Chapter objective two may be used to stimulate application of ethical principles into students' management perspectives.

Objective 2: Give one example of a nursing care or nursing management decision derived from each of the following ethical principles:

a. Respect for personhood
b. Autonomy
c. Justice
d. Veracity

Time: 15-20 minutes plus follow up discussion

Ask students to give 1 or 2 examples of nursing management decision derived from the assigned ethical principle.

Divide class into four groups. Assign one of the four above ethical principles to each group.

Reconvene class and have each group share examples.

TEST QUESTIONS

KNOWLEDGE AND COMPREHENSION

True : False

T F 20.01. Veracity is the basis for a patient's hope of benefit from nursing services.

T F 20.02. The principle of nonmaleficence allows passive euthanasia by caregivers of terminally ill patients.

T F 20.03. Kant's fundamental principle is that one should act only on that maxim which you can intend should become a universal law.

Multiple Choice

20.04. Which of the following are criteria which should be used when several ethical theories apply to the same situation?
- a. look for the degree of internal consistency
- b. identify the extent to which implications of the theory agree with personal experiences of morality
- c. look for the extent the theory provides guidance in the situation
- d. all of above

20.05. The ANA Code of Ethics for Nurses includes statements regarding:
- a. patient's right to privacy
- b. maintaining competency in nursing
- c. respect for human dignity
- d. all of above

Matching: Match the term to the definition by placing the correct letter in the space provided.

	Definition	Term
____	20.06. fundamental fact, rule, law	a. attitude
____	20.07. deeply held preference, interest	b. belief
____	20.08. general meaning of a phenomenon	c. concept
____	20.09. opinion	d. principle
____	20.10. organized set of interrelated facts or rules	e. theory
		f. value
____	20.11. firm conviction	

APPLICATION, ANALYSIS, AND/OR SYNTHESIS

True : False

T F 20.12. After studying ethics, you and your staff will make the same decisions in a difficult patient care situation.

Multiple Choice

20.13. The stressed nurse applied wrist restraints to the confused patient even though a family member said he would stay with the patient until the patient settled down. The nurse may be practicing:
a. occurrent coercion
b. fidelity
c. justice
d. liberty of action

20.14. The nurse who shares information about home care options for the discharged stroke patient, but withholds information about nursing home placement is:
a. beneficent
b. limiting patient autonomy
c. cognizant of nonmaleficence
d. practicing dispositional coercion

20.15. The nurse gave an emergency pre op laminectomy patient IM valium and pain medication. Later the nurse discovered the patient had not yet signed the pre op consent form. She then took the form to the patient who signed. The patient is paralyzed postoperatively. The patient's family is encouraging him to sue.
Grounds for the suit could include.
a. the nurse did not properly care for the patient
b. surgery was not performed in a timely manner
c. the patient did not give informed consent
d. all of above

20.16. The nurse who limits time spent in caring for an elderly stroke patient in order to have more time to care for a twenty year old paraplegic is:
a. practicing implicit rationing
b. is using age as a rationing criteria
c. is valuing youth
d. all of above

20.17. If the nurse is practicing Kant's categorical imperative, which of the following could she do?
a. administer a placebo
b. persistently encourage the person to participate in biomedical research
c. tell the patient his real diagnosis when asked
d. all of above

Matching: Match the moral principle practiced in each of the nursing situations below by placing the appropriate letter in the space provided.

Nursing practices

____ 20.18. The nurse asks patient which pain medication he refers.

____ 20.19. The nurse arranged for the family to have dinner with the patient.

____ 20.20. The nurse waited for two additional helpers to move the patient to the stretcher.

____ 20.21. The patient asked what the medication was for. The nurse explained the purpose of the medication.

____ 20.22. The nurse followed through with her promise to get a list of home care resources.

____ 20.23. A neighbor asked what was wrong with a mutual friend who is hospitalized. The nurse did not answer.

____ 20.24. The nurse administrator tried to practice staff:patient ratios according to established criteria on each of the units.

Moral Principles

a. beneficence

b. confidentiality

c. facilitate autonomy

d. fidelity

e. justice

f. nonmaleficence

g. veracity

Matching: Match the term to the example to which it applies by placing the appropriate letter in the space provided.

	Example	Term
____	20.25. The nurse believes that the patient cannot help behaving that way.	a. deception
____	20.26. The patient has the free will to choose the treatment that will be appropriate for him.	b. determinists
____	20.27. The nurse diverted the terminally ill patient's attention to the progress he had made.	c. libertarians
____	20.28. The senior nurse may choose holiday off preference according to personnel policy.	d. normative ethics
____	20.29. The study was to determine the best approach for deciding the nursing action that should be taken.	e. right
____	20.30. The nurse debated which patient would benefit most by her spending the last 20 minutes with him.	f. utilitarianism

ANSWERS	TEXT REFERENCE
20.01. T	p. 369
20.02. F	p. 371
20.03. T	p. 373
20.04. d	p. 372
20.05. d	p. 375
20.06. d	p. 366
20.07. f	p. 366
20.08. c	p. 366
20.09. a	p. 366
20.10. e	p. 367
20.11. b	p. 367
20.12. F	p. 367
20.13. a	p. 368
20.14. b	p. 367, 368
20.15. c	p. 382
20.16. d	p. 378+
20.17. c	p. 373
20.18. c	p. 367
20.19. a	p. 367, 371
20.20. f	p. 367, 371
20.21. g	p. 367, 368, 369
20.22. d	p. 367, 371, 372
20.23. b	p. 367, 372
20.24. e	p. 367, 370
20.25. b	p. 368
20.26. c	p. 368
20.27. a	p. 370
20.28. e	p. 371
20.29. d	p. 372
20.30. f	p. 373

CHAPTER

21

Obtaining and Using Power

Nurses are hesitant to grasp the benefits and legitimacy of seeking power. All too often the concept of power is perceived negatively. To promote power awareness and legitimacy students need to take a look at all aspects of power. The text content and the activities presented in this *Manual* will assist faculty in conveying that needed awareness of power. The aware student can then proceed to use power as a positive force.

KEY TERMS

compensatory power
condign power
conditioned power
expert power
integrative power
nutrient power
position power
power
referent power
scapegoat
social power
synergic power

OUTLINE

I. Introduction
   A. Power defined
   B. Differing orientations re. power
II. Types of power
   A. Sources of power
      1. Personal
      2. Positional
      3. Structural
         a. Job description
         b. Chain of command
         c. Centrality
         d. Specialization
         e. Formalization
         f. Committees
      4. Social
      5. Expert
   B. Actual or potential
   C. Direct or indirect
   D. Benevolent or destructive
      1. Nutrient power
      2. Integrative power
   E. Legitimate or illegitimate
   F. Unilateral or bilateral
   G. Synergic power
   H. Exertion of power
      1. Influence
      2. Manipulative
      3. Competitive
      4. Exploitive

I. Role of control

III. Power instrumentalities and sources
   A. Condign power
      1. Described
      2. Relationship to organization
   B. Compensatory power
      1. Described
      2. Relationship to conditional power
   C. Conditioned power

IV. Reasons for acquiring power

V. Manifestations of power
   A. Five levels of power
      1. Power to be
      2. Power of self-affirmation
      3. Power of self-assertion
      4. Power of aggression
      5. Power of violence
   B. Power-oriented characteristics
      1. Concern for personal impact vs. performance quality
      2. Chooses status-oriented and competitive situations
   C. Democratic perspective
   D. Power and the hierarchy
      1. Bureaucracy
      2. Decentralization

VI. Power principles
   A. Power is dynamic and elusive
   B. Power is actively acquired
   C. Any means may be used to acquire control
   D. Winning requires total commitment to goals
   E. Restraint ensures effective power use
   F. Power relationships are highly situational
   G. Power has spatial dimensions
   H. Employees desire clear definitions of power and control relationships

VII. Skills used in power acquisition
   A. Peer skills
   B. Leadership skills
   C. Information processing skills
   D. Conflict resolution skills
   E. Skill in unstructured decision making
   F. Entrepreneurial skills

VIII. Exertion and use of power
   A. Unity between self and followers
      1. Active listening to subordinates
      2. Application or withholding of punishment
      3. Selective granting of rewards
      4. Channeling information
   B. Overcoming faction power
   C. Use of hiring, firing, retiring, promoting, and disciplining
      1. Scapegoat
      2. Power examples
   D. Using spatial aspects for gaining control
   E. Money as power symbol
   F. Quit position while ahead
   G. Effective time use
      1. Status interactions
      2. Time as a tool to control others
      3. Limited accessibility to others
      4. Avoid open confrontations
      5. Desensitize self to uncertainties
   H. Use of committees
      1. Control of committee agenda
      2. Control of committee composition
   I. Use of communication channels
      1. Selectively distribute information
      2. Selectively enhance staff in development
   J. Territorial claim
      1. Lower floor
      2. Corner office
      3. Space use
      4. Color-design boundaries
   K. Use of own office
   L. Use of space of powerful other
   M. Telephone usage
      1. Taking calls
      2. Holding calls
      3. Initiating calls
   N. Verbal and nonverbal language
   O. Extraordinary performance
      1. Visibility
      2. Activity span
   P. Timing arrival
   Q. Use of outsider to present different position
   R. Use of recording during meeting
      1. Tape recorder
      2. Own notes on legal pad
      3. Avoid secretarial role
   S. Public relations campaign

IX. Summary

CLASS OR HOMEWORK ACTIVITY: Power Self-Study Sheets

The Power Self-Study Sheets presented as Figure 21.1 (at the end of this *Manual*) can be assigned as homework, or completed during class as controlled notes, or by assigning to groups of three during class. A group approach to the study of power is recommended as it promotes interstudent discussion of power and promotes the perception of power as a potentially positive rather than a negative tool. By involving students in presentation of material, the faculty is deflecting the negative reaction to power from him/herself to student groups. As the student groups work through the material, many of the negative perceptions of power will be resolved.

DISCUSSION IDEAS: Power

Chapter objectives 1, 3, 4, and 5 may each be used as discussion topics. Objectives 3, 4, and 5 are most suitable for RN to BSN students and graduate nursing students. Objective 1 may appropriately be used with all levels of nursing students.

Objective 1: Describe situations in which a nurse manger should employ personal power, position power, expert power, and referent power to achieve a social good.

Objective 3: Describe the behavior used by your nurse manager to acquire power advantage over another in the health agency.

Objective 4: Describe one way in which your manager manipulates spatial cues to acquire a greater amount of power than other nurse managers.

Objective 5: Describe one situation in which your nurse manager timed an agency event so as to achieve power advantage over an employee.

GROUP ACTIVITY: Managing the problem nurse manager

The group activity will involve the issues contained in chapter objectives 1, 2, 3, and 4.

Objective 1: Describe situations in which a nurse manager should employ personal power, position power, expert power, and referent power to achieve a social good.

Objective 2: Describe three behaviors that would indicate strong needs for power.

Objective 3: Describe the behavior used by your nurse manager to acquire power advantage over another in the health agency.

Objective 4: Describe one way in which your manager manipulates spatial cues to acquire a greater amount of power than other nurse managers.

Situation

In Hospital Y nursing management practices, policies, and procedures are outdated by several years. The nursing division is making only spotty progress in updating nursing managerial and administrative approaches. Although decentralization and participatory management are institutional goals, management decisions are rarely delegated downward beyond the Assistant Director of Nursing (ADON).

Administrative Profiles

CEO practices a global perspective in regard to the facility. He practices delegation in expecting divisional directors to be responsible for their divisions. He practices priorities of money management, strategic planning, and catch-up in relation to competitive facilities. Frequently he must "put out fires" involving medical personnel and competitive physicians. He is struggling to gain a current institutional posture. He spends considerable time outside the institution.

The second in command is newer in his position. His focus is on day-to-day and fiscal operations. The current major project is the updating of the data information systems. He is working long hours and becoming more and more isolated.

The Nurse Administrator is a long-term employee and is very loyal to the facility. She is looking toward retirement. She is a bright, pleasant person who is kindly and motherly toward her subordinates.

The ADON, around whom the assignment centers, is a congenial, pleasant, and soft-spoken person. She is not found actively involved in employee conflicts, but rather gives directives in a soft-spoken, congenial manner. She has befriended nurse union activists and is perceived to be their ally. When questioned why a particular thing is still done in the "old way," her response is likely to be, "Oh, I wouldn't dream of touching that. You know how the union would respond." Scheduling preferences are granted to a select few. Institutional loyalty is strong. She frequently keeps others waiting seated in the hallway for meetings. Meetings are usually conducted in her office which is beyond the desks of several supportive staff. She convenes committees of which she need not be a part.

Activities

Assessment

1. From the above profiles identify both positive and negative examples of:

    - positional power
    - personal power
    - structural power
    - social power

    (The examples may indicate what is being practiced or what is not being practiced and should be.)

2. Which ADON behaviors indicate a strong need for power?

3. Which ADON behaviors indicate a pursuit for more power?

4. From the above profiles state a spatial cue for power exhibited by the ADON

Problem/Need

The challenge is to either (1) grow the ADON into practicing her role differently to promote rather than stop participative management and updating, or (2) to facilitate the ADON's resignation.

Planning

1. Given the above assessment and power information you have learned, what would you recommend in an effort to upgrade the ADON's practice of her role?

2. Assume that the above plan did not produce a change, but rather the ADON has become even more controlling. What strategies could be implemented to facilitate the ADON's resignation? Do seek to strive for a win-win or at least a win-"save face" approach.

TEST QUESTIONS

KNOWLEDGE AND COMPREHENSION

True : False

T F 21.01. Power is neither inherently good or bad.

T F 21.02. Personal power is proportional to strength of the manger's self concept and self esteem.

T F 21.03. As decentralization increases, the power of first line managers decreases.

T F 21.04. A nurse manager with need for power will also display high achievement.

T F 21.05. Use of manipulative power to control professional nurses is inappropriate use of power.

T F 21.06. Without power the nurse manager cannot compete for scarce resources.

T F 21.07. To retain power the manager must actively pursue power.

T F 21.08. To win in the game of organizational politics the manager must be totally committed to personal goals.

T F 21.09. Forcing an employee's retirement is as powerful an act as firing the employee.

Multiple Choice

21.10. The manager who gives compensatory time as a reward for extensive committee work is practicing:
a. social power
b. direct power
c. expert power
d. integrative power

21.11. Which of the following is a listing of the levels of power potential by increasing intensity?
a. self-affirmation, aggression, to be, self-assertion, violence
b. to be, self-assertion, aggression, se;f-affirmation, violence
c. to be, self-affirmation, self-assertion, aggression, violence
d. none of the above

21.12. The power oriented manager will:
a. welcome employees who make impromptu office visits
b. ask the secretary to take phone messages
c. attend only meetings pertaining to current priorities
d. all of above

APPLICATION, ANALYSIS, AND/OR SYNTHESIS

Matching: Match the type of power to the behavior by placing the letter in the space provided.

		Behavior	Type of Power
___	21.13.	the nurse manager attends hospital sponsored activities such as open house, Christmas party, and the bowling games	a. expert
			b. illegitimate
___	21.14.	the nurse manager encourages the staff nurse to pursue her BSN degree	c. integrative
			d. legitimate
___	21.15.	the nurse unit manager arranges the staffing schedule so she will not have to work with a difficult RN	e. nutrient
			f. personal
___	21.16.	the nurses followed the guidance of the nurse manager because of her knowledge	g. positional
___	21.17.	the unit manager power level is the same regardless of who holds the position	h. social
___	21.18.	the unit manager had the confidence to confront two feuding employees	
___	21.19.	The nurse administrator worked with the mental health unit to devise a proposal for an employee assistance program, and presented the proposal to the hospital administrator.	

Multiple Choice

21.20. As a nurse manager you prefer to use *positional* power in contrast to personal power. Which of the following would be (an) example(s) of direct positional power?
  a. You ask Mrs. Gobetween, RN, to have Mr. Sluffman, RN, complete a task.
  b. You schedule part-time Mrs. Problemchile, RN, only on the evening weekend shifts.
  c. You establish a policy of advanced placement and salary increases for persons showing advanced merit in clinical practice.
  d. all of above

21.21. Which of the following behaviors is indicative of behavior demonstrating a need for power or control?
  a. Committee member Imhere arrives early and focuses discussion on agenda item
  b. Nursing Assistant Howto asks her mentor how to do a task
  c. New Nurse Ready completes the orientation skills demonstrations early
  d. Nurse Unit Manager FaCilitate completes an assigned report and submits it to administration on time

21.22. Which of the following demonstrates increase of power through the use of spatial aspects?
a. the nursing office is relocated to the administrative wing
b. the nursing administrator moves files and the nursing secretary into an empty room across the hall
c. the nursing administrator places chairs in the hallway for persons waiting to see her
d. all of above

21.23. During downsizing the hospital laid off nurses. Patient care needs later increased requiring rehiring. The union contract required that the rehiring be based upon "seniority." A position opened in ICU. Nurse Oldtimer, the senior laid-off nurse, is without ICU experience but is hired. ICU nurses notify the nurse manager that they are filing a grievance to get rid of Nurse Oldtimer. How might the nurse manager apply power theory and turn this situation into a potentially positive direction?
a. The nurse manager reassures the nursing staff that Nurse Oldtimer is a capable nurse and will soon learn.
b. The nurse manager meets with the concerned staff and Nurse Oldtimer, shares the contract requirements, and asks them what should be done?
c. The nurse manager provides extra staff development activities for Nurse Oldtimer.
d. The nurse manager transfers Nurse Oldtimer to another unit, and hires an experienced new nurse.

21.24. Which of the following communication examples demonstrates power seeking?
a. The manager turned the discussion into a debate.
b. The manager called a meeting to ask for input regarding an area of patient complaint.
c. The manager chatted informally at lunch with the secretarial staff.
d. all of above

21.25. The assistant director of nursing no longer fulfills her duties well. Which of the following actions might the wise administrator take to speed the assistant director of nursing's retirement?
a. allow committees to make decision previously made by the assistant director of nursing
b. assign mundane work to the assistant director of nursing
c. encourage the assistant director of nursing to talk about the past
d. all of above

21.26. A good time for the power conscious manager to resign would be after:
a. resolving a pervasive problem
b. being awarded a coveted honor
c. delivering seminars for a recognized national professional organization
d. all of above

ANSWERS	TEXT REFERENCE
21.01. T	p. 387
21.02. T	p. 387
21.03. F	p. 392
21.04. F	p. 391
21.05. T	p. 390
21.06. T	p. 391
21.07. T	p. 392
21.08. F	p. 393
21.09. T	p. 394
21.10. b	p. 389
21.11. c	p. 391
21.12. b	p. 397
21.13. h	p. 388
21.14. e	p. 389
21.15. b	p. 389
21.16. a	p. 388
21.17. g	p. 387
21.18. f	p. 387
21.19. c	p. 388
21.20. c	p. 387, 388
21.21. a	p. 398
21.22. d	p. 396
21.23. b	p. 398
21.24. a	p. 392
21.25. d	p. 395
21.26. d	p. 395

CHAPTER

22

Problem Solving

Experienced nurses will quickly value the exploration of problem solving presented. Constructive problem solving guidelines and tools are presented from assessing a situation and identifying root causes to promoting characteristics in self and others that lead to good quality problem resolution. Students at all levels will enjoy the chapter group activities as they explore problem solving with Nurse Naivette and Topseyturvey Hospital.

KEY TERMS

convergent thinking
deductive thinking
divergent thinking
double loop learning
free association
inductive inference
inference
problem
single loop learning

OUTLINE

I. Overview
   A. Definition
   B. Types of problems
   C. Significance of problem solving

II. Problem solving methods
   A. Trial and error
      1. Defined
      2. Limitation
   B. Scientific experimentation
      1. Defined
      2. Use
      3. Limitations
   C. Critique
      1. Defined
      2. Process
   D. Metaphor-based free association
      1. Process
      2. Manager's abilities
         a. Previous work experience
         b. Analytical thinking
         c. Creative thinking
         d. Inductive thinking
         e. Deductive thinking
      3. Essential analyses
         a. Problem situation
         b. Subject's dissatisfaction

III. Principles of problem solving
   A. Principles
      1. Separate large from small problems
      2. Delegate smaller problems
      3. Consult with experts for difficult problems

4. Avoid crisis decisions for better quality resolutions
5. Perfection is impossible

B. Promote subordinate problem solving
1. Include problem-solving responsibilities in job descriptions and performance evaluations
2. Provide problem-solving instruction to subordinates
a. "In basket" exercises
b. Group approach
c. Utilize problem solving frame work

IV. Encouraging problem-solving behavior
A. Prompt rewards
B. Use of incentives
C. Facilitating climate
D. Problems in promoting problem solving

V. Characteristics of skillful problem solvers
A. High subject expertise
B. High creativity
C. Wide range of knowledge
D. Competence in scientific inquiry
E. Differing problem solving approaches
1. Serial approach to problems
2. Prioritize problems
3. Concurrent problems
4. Branching problems

VI. Group decision making
A. Advantages of
B. Principles of
C. Participatory management systems
1. Impact of
2. Promotion of
3. Role of facilitator

VII. Focus groups
A. History
B. Description
C. Use
D. Phases
1. Surveys
2. Administrative input
3. Conduct
E. Examples

VIII. Definitions
A. Divergent thinking
B. Convergent thinking
C. Decision making
D. Inference
E. Inductive inference

IX. Steps of problem solving
A. Steps of problem critique
1. Problem definition
a. Identify problem consequences
b. Identify subproblems
2. Data collection
a. Identify needed data
b. Identify likely data sources
c. Specify data collecting methods
3. Possible solutions
a. Saturate self with information
b. Explore differing perspectives
c. Allow "incubation" time
d. Refine "crazy" solutions
4. Selection of solution
a. Identify needed concrete changes
b. Determine criteria for satisfactory resolution
c. Predict consequences of changes
d. Identify pros and cons of options
5. Implementation of preferred solution
6. Evaluation
a. Assess process and product
b. Effect of solution
7. Example of focus group problem solving
a. Five process criteria
b. Nine problem solving steps

B. Types of problems
1. Problems of simplicity
2. Problems of disordered complexity
3. Problems of organized complexity

C. Defining the problem and collecting data
1. Purpose of problem definition
2. Separate root cause from symptomatic problems
a. Identify differences when desired goal is achieved and when it is not
b. Apply negative thinking to rule out potential root causes
3. Gather information for problem definition
a. Gather problem oriented information
b. Interviewing guidelines
4. Single-loop learning
5. Double-loop learning

6. Examination of situation

D. Generating solutions
   1. Identify agency's highest priority goals
   2. Generate multiple options
   4. Idea generation checklists
   5. Psychodrama
   6. Brainstorming
   7. Synectics
   8. Pareto analysis
      a. Description
      b. Process
         (1). Possible causes
         (2). Histogram

E. Selecting a solution
   1. Rate against stated criteria
   2. Criteria examples
   3. Identification of preferred solution

X. Summary

GROUP ACTIVITIES: Problem Solving: Nurse Naivette and Topseyturvey Hospital's Outpatient Surgery Diagnostic Center

Faculty may choose to use just one, all, or a combination of the activities.

Time: The time to carry out each objective is stated.

Preparation: In advance of class reproduce a copy of the situation for each group.

Situation: Nurse Naivette and Topseyturvey Hospital's reorganized outpatient surgery and diagnostic center.

February: At Topseyturvey Hospital finances are extremely tight. Administrative response is more reorganization of services and staff.

Nurse Naivette, a competent operating room staff nurse, is hired to reorganize the physical facility and operations to combine existing outpatient surgery and existing and new diagnostic services into one center. Nurse Naivette is flattered by being offered the position and enthusiastically accepts. Nurse unit managers at Hospital Topseyturvey are responsible for unit budget, staff allocation, service recommendations, as well as the overall day-to-day operations. Administration also requires quarterly reports of program services, and recommendations, and monthly variance reports.

Physicians opposed the administrative plan to combine the services but now begrudgingly acknowledge the idea might be good.

June: Nurse Naivette calls in sick. She has been working ten-hour days, frequently taking work home. On Tuesday administration called to remind her that the quarterly report was delinquent and a variance report was due. She was given three days grace to submit the reports. In addition administration asked for a proposed biennium budget. When she questioned that this was due in three days, administration reminded her that both the variance and quarterly reports were overdue. Administration stated that she had been working on the project for more than four months, that surely she had a good feel for costs by now and could pull together a budget proposal.

Thursday: Nurse Naivette snapped at the housekeeper who came along with the vacuum cleaner.

Nurse Naivette closeted herself Wednesday and Thursday refusing to answer the phone or knocks on the door. Since she believes wholeheartedly in the Outpatient surgery and diagnostic center, and recognizes administrative concern over finances, she conscientiously wrote a detailed variance report and a budget proposal which included only minor remodeling of the chosen area, a very conservative (but incomplete) biennial budget, and staffing allocation.

The reports were submitted to administration on Friday at 5:00 pm, but administration was already gone.

Monday: Nurse Naivette receives a rather snippy memo from personnel saying "since we were unable to reach you, I've gone ahead and written the position description for the Surgi-center nurses. I hope you are happy with the content. I've also posted the positions in-house."

Nurse Naivette was not happy. The position description was based on outmoded performance expectancies.

July: Nurse Naivette was hired as Nurse Unit Manager of the Outpatient Surgery and Diagnostic Center. She was to outfit and set up the unit, obtain needed equipment and supplies, and interview applicants in conjunction with the personnel office.

Personnel scheduled applicant interviews. The interviews were conducted. Personnel and Nurse Naivette disagreed about the qualifications of one applicant. The personnel person responded "but she meets the position description requirements."

July 15: Diagnostic services were shifted to Nurse Naivette's new area. Nurse Naivette received a complaint from two physicians the first week that staff did not know how to operate equipment.

August: Outpatient surgery is transferred to the newly organized unit.

June Next Year: Nurse Naivette is called into the Administrator's office.

- The Outpatient Surgery and Diagnostic Center is running at a loss. Why?
- The physicians would like to add a laser specialty unit. Administration thinks that the perfect place to put it is the Outpatient Surgery and Diagnostic Center. What does Nurse Naivette think about the idea?

Three days later: Nurse Naivette is absent.

Activity I: Problem identification

Objective 3: Use the technique of Pareto Analysis to identify one or two principal causes of a multi-causal problem.

Time 30 minutes

Assignment: Using Pareto Analysis

- identify as many causes for the problems as possible
- identify relative importance of each causative factor
- which are the two or three most important causes?

Activity II: Classifying Problems

Objective 2: Identify one problem of the following types: a. Problem of simplicity; b. Problem of disordered complexity; c. Problem of ordered complexity.

Time: 15 minutes

Assignment: Using problems identified above:

- identify a problem of simplicity
- identify a problem of disordered complexity
- Identify a problem of ordered complexity

Activity III: Identifying root causes

Time: 30 minutes

Assignment:

1. Identify the *root cause(s)* of the problem of simplicity that the group identified above.
2. What manifestations have occurred related to the problem?
3. If the identified root cause(s) is/are not corrected, what will be the future effect on:
   - Nurse Naivette?
   - the combined Outpatient Surgery and Diagnostic Center?
   - Hospital Topseyturvey?

Activity IV: Problem-solving options

Faculty: You might choose to have one group of students pursue problem solutions through Activity IV, and another group utilize Activity V.

Time: 30 minutes

1. On the basis of the above assessments, generate two possible solutions for the problem.

Activity V: Using a checklist as a tool to identify problem solutions

Develop an ideas checklist to identify three additional (less obvious) possible solutions to the identified problem.

Time: 1 class period

Assignment:

1. Utilizing the concepts presented under "Idea Checklists" (text, page 412) adapt the text questions and create at least three additional questions that will stimulate the group to discover novel solutions.

2. Apply the "checklist" to the situation and strive to discover (a) novel solution(s) which is/are not obvious solutions. State the novel solution(s).

3. Consider the solution options created by the group under Activity III, and the novel solution(s) the group has just discovered. Is there an even better solution that incorporates various aspects of a combination of these solutions?

4. State the preferred solution.

CLASS ACTIVITY: Brainstorming

Time 45 minutes

Preparation: To be most effective, the group should be told the topic 24 to 48 hours in advance.

Possible topics: What nursing services could be identified as product lines in a given health agency? One group might focus on an acute care hospital, another on a long-term care facility, another on a home care agency, another on a county health department.

Introduction: The purpose of brainstorming is to break through conventional thinking to rapidly generate many ideas. Emphasis is on the number of ideas. No idea is too bizarre. Every idea is accepted **nonjudgementally**. Usually a group will respond with many ideas followed by a lull. When the lull occurs the group is to be encouraged to identify additional ideas. Some of the best ideas will be suggested at this time.

Process:

Divide into groups of 10-12 members.
Set a time limit for the generation of ideas.
Identify a group leader to record ideas. Reminder, the group leader is to record all ideas. No judgment of ideas is to be made.
The group then reviews the ideas generated to identify those which are new ideas, and to consider the flexibility of the ideas.
The new ideas should be set aside for later refinement and/or development.
Two days after the brainstorming session the group leader should contact group members for any additional ideas since the brainstorming session.

Objective 1: Describe manner in which divergent and convergent thinking are used in problem solving.

Identify times during the brainstorming activities when

- divergent thinking occurred, and
- convergent thinking occurred.

TEST QUESTIONS

KNOWLEDGE AND COMPREHENSION

True : False

T F 22.01. A systematic approach to problem solving increases organizational productivity.

T F 22.02. To solve a problem through critique, a manager must promote effected employees' dissatisfaction with the situation.

T F 22.03. Adults learn best through immediate application and experimentation.

T F 22.04. A hostile climate inhibits problem solving while a soft climate stimulates creative problem solving.

T F 22.05. Trial and error is the problem-solving method most often used by nurse managers.

T F 22.06. The most critical step in the problem-solving process is the solution.

T F 22.07. Problems are most apt to develop in complex nursing situations.

T F 22.08. Weighing all relevant evidence is necessary to identify a workable problem solution.

Multiple Choice

22.09. Problem resolution usually requires:
a. application of existing policies
b. new knowledge or skills, or attitudes
c. a new combination of existing ideas and abilities
d. a combination of a and b

22.10. Which of the following problem-solving methods would be *AVOIDED* by a nurse administrator who is valuing time use?
a. trial and error
b. scientific method
c. critique
d. metaphor-based techniques

22.11. Ethical consideration, control costs and patient suffering limit the use of which of the problem solving methods?
a. trial and error
b. scientific method
c. critique
d. metaphor-based techniques

22.12. Smaller problems should be resolved through:
a. committee
b. administration
c. policy
d. organizational restructuring

Matching: Match the term to the appropriate description by placing letter in space provided. *Each answer may NOT be used.*

		Description	Term
___	22.13.	A provocative situation for which a person has no ready response.	a. convergent
___	22.14.	Thinking that progresses from individual items to the whole.	b. deductive
___	22.15.	Consumer group discusses a specified service.	c. devergent
___	22.16.	Thinking in which several problem solutions are generated.	d. double loop
___	22.17.	Thinking in which one solution is selected from several options.	e. focus
___	22.18.	A judgement is made which goes beyond given data.	f. inductive
___	22.19.	When both the employee and the manager observe a problem procedure and share observations, they are practicing _?_ learning.	g. inference
___	22.20.	One or a few problem cause(s) is/are responsible for most problem occurrences.	h. Pareto analysis
			i. problem

APPLICATION, ANALYSIS, AND/OR SYNTHESIS

Matching: Match the Problem Type to the related Situation by placing the letter in the space provided.

	Situation	Problem Type
___ 22.21.	To project a biennium budget for the new Surgi-center, Nurse Naivette needs to forecast the number and types of surgeries per day, month, and year.	a. Problem of simplicity b. Problem of disordered complexity c. Problem of organized complexity
___ 22.22.	Staffing of the new Surgi-center, outpatient surgery, and inpatient surgery services will be done through pooling the OR staff and deploying them per need.	
___ 22.23.	When scrub nurse Howtodoit is on, average patient anesthesia time per surgery type is less.	

Multiple Choice

22.24. Which of the following are key characteristics of the nurse manager who is a skillful problem solver?
a. the nurse manager delegates smaller problems which can be resolved through existing policy.
b. the nurse manager includes the involved individuals in problem solving
c. the nurse manager practices various types of highly creative thinking
d. all of above

22.25. The unit manager worked conscientiously to improve a quality deficiency. The next review demonstrated considerable improvement. Which of the following nurse administrator responses will contribute to resolution of other problems by the unit managers?
a. place unit managers on the quality management committee
b. request review of the same patient problem three months from the last review
c. take unit managers to lunch in recognition of their success
d. all of above

22.26. The group could not agree on what the real problem was. Because of time constraints and group cohesiveness, the group devised three solution to the problem. The likely outcome will be:
a. the original problem well recycle
b. one of the solutions will work
c. the group will feel self-fulfilled in completing task on time
d. the group will be ineffective in the future

22.27. Which of the following are behaviors of a facilitative group leader?
a. Nurse Leadon conducts meeting in a manner that encourages participation of each committee member.
b. Nurse Leadon clarifies a member suggestion by sharing additional data.
c. Nurse Leadon gave her opinion regarding the problem when asked.
d. all of above

22.28. The committee worked hard to identify the root problem. Nurse Leadon then deferred exploring solution to the next meeting.

a. Nurse Leadon's behavior will dampen the momentum of problem resolution.
b. Committee members will more likely identify creative solutions.
c. Nurse Leadon will review the problem to devise a solution to present at the next meeting.
d. all of above

22.29. The outpatient mental health services redesigned their therapy program in response to recurring patient problems. For a short time the identified patient problems were reduced. Six months later the identified patient problems are reoccurring frequently. Which of the following most likely represents what is actually occurring?

a. the redesigned therapy program is not being carried out appropriately
b. the root causes of the patient problems were not identified
c. the current patient population is a very needy group which is resistive to therapy
d. staff do not understand the new therapy program and/or lack the skills and knowledge to carry out the new program

22.30. Which of the following will facilitate selection of the most promising problem solution?

a. compare each solution against the same desired criteria
b. try each solution for a designated period of time to determine which provides the best results
c. choose the solution with the broadest scope to cover more bases
d. all of above

ANSWERS	TEXT REFERENCE
22.01. T	p. 402
22.02. T	p. 403
22.03. T	p. 404
22.04. F	p. 404
22.05. F	p. 408
22.06. F	p. 408
22.07. T	p. 411
22.08. F	p. 409
22.09. c	p. 401
22.10. a	p. 402
22.11. b	p. 402
22.12. c	p. 403, 404
22.13. i	p. 401
22.14. f	p. 403
22.15. e	p. 406, 407
22.16. c	p. 407
22.17. a	p. 407, 408
22.18. g	p. 408
22.19. d	p. 411
22.20. h	p. 414
22.21. b	p. 409
22.22. c	p. 409
22.23. a	p. 409
22.24. d	p. 403
22.25. c	p. 404
22.26. a	p. 406
22.27. d	p. 406
22.28. b	p. 409
22.29. b	p. 409
22.30. a	p. 414

CHAPTER

23

Decision Making

Decision making is crucial to the leadership ability of the nurse manager. This chapter helps the student to understand theoretical perspectives of decision making, and arms the student with a repertoire of decision-making strategies and decision-making aids.

KEY TERMS

administrative man	mixed scanning
chameon strategy	normative model
defensive avoidance	omissions
descriptive model	opportunistic
economic man	optimizing
hypervigilant	overload
maximax strategy	queuing
maximin strategy	satisficing
mini-regret strategy	strategic decisions

OUTLINE

I. Overview
  A. Importance of decision making
  B. Increased complexity of decision making
    1. Information quantity
    2. Participative management practices
    3. Need for high-level communication skills
  C. Increased need for high-quality decisions

II. Decision making defined
  A. Definition of decision making
  B. Definition of decision-making process
  C. Placement of decision making in problem solving
  D. Characteristics of good decision making
    1. Decisions are timely
    2. Decisions are based on clinical reality
    3. Decisions must lead to wise use of resources
    4. Decisions must be communicated to motivate
  E. Approaches to decision making
    1. Economic man (ideal)
    2. Administrative man (pragmatic)

- F. Historical placement of decision
- G. Generate other decisions
- H. Decision quality dependent upon information quality and quantity

III. Information overload
- A. Defined
- B. Negative results
  1. Errors
  2. Omissions
  3. Queuing
  4. Filtering
  5. Manager-stressed responses
     a. Approximation actions
     b. Avoidance
     c. Flee workplace
- C. Positive responses
  1. Classify information
  2. Delegate

IV. Decisional conflict
- A. Psychological stress
- B. Coping techniques
  1. Unconflicted inertia
  2. Unconflicted change
  3. Defensive avoidance
  4. Hypervigilance
  5. Vigilance

V. Uncertainty and risk
- A. Need for differentiation
  1. Definitions
  2. Choice
- B. Ignorance and error
  1. Definitions
  2. Input generalization

VI. Types of decisions
- A. Decision types
  1. Strategic
  2. Administrative
  3. Operational
- B. Decision classification
  1. Programmed
  2. Nonprogrammed
- C. Decision mode
  1. Normative or ideal
  2. Descriptive

VII. Decision strategy
- A. Definition
- B. Decision making strategies
- C. Questions for determining most appropriate strategy
- D. Explication of strategies
  1. Optimizing
  2. Satisficing
  3. Opportunistic
  4. Do nothing
  5. Identify and remove critical limiting factor
  6. Maximax
  7. Maximin
  8. Mini-regret
  9. Precautionary
  10. Evolutionary
  11. Chameon
- E. Psychological influences on decision making style
  1. Four dimensions by Jung
     a. Perception
     b. Judgment
     c. Attitudes toward life
     d. Attitudes toward outer world
  2. Polarization
  3. Myers Briggs Type Indicator

VIII. Steps of decision making
- A. Steps described
  1. Determine agency goals and priorities
  2. Perceive need for a decision
  3. Identify criteria for successful response
  4. Identify alternative courses of action
  5. Weighing alternatives
  6. Select one alternative
  7. Commit to action
  8. Implement decision
  9. Adherence to decision
- B. Importance of each step (1-9)
- C. Group responses to steps

IX. "Root" and "branch" approaches to decision making
- A. "Root" approach to decision making described
- B. "Branch" approach to decision making described

X. Aids to decision making
- A. Models
- B. Games
- C. Decision tree
- D. Cause and effect fishbone diagram
  1. Description
  2. Examples
- E. Brainstorming
- F. Nominal group process
- G. Delphi method
- H. Fishbowling
- I. Decision analysis

XI. Individual vs. group decision making

- A. Reasons for leader-made decisions
- B. Reasons for group-made decisions
- C. Disadvantages of group decisions
- D. Promoting group effectiveness
- E. Negotiated decision making
  1. Phases of
  2. Study example

XII. Methods of decision making
- A. Vroom and Yetton model
  1. Five methods of decision making
     - a. Autocratic I
     - b. Autocratic II
     - c. Consultive I
     - d. Consultive II
     - e. Group II
  2. Seven variables to identify "best" method
  3. Six rules for use of the Vroom and Yetton model
  4. Updated model
- B. Study example

XIII. Summary

DISCUSSION IDEA: Information Overload

Objective 2: Describe a nursing situation in which information overload prevented you from making an effective clinical or management decision.

The above objective is appropriate for RN to BSN and graduate students. By adapting the objective to include a poor quality decision made in the role of student, all levels of students may identify with the problem of information overload.

Questions

1. Describe how information overload made you feel?
2. Describe your decision response.
3. Given the same situation, how would you like to respond?

DISCUSSION IDEA: Risk and uncertainty in decision making

Preparation: Obtain a position advertisement or posting which might be of interest to the students.

Activity

1. Present an advertisement or position posting to the students. Ask students to decide whether they would apply or not.
2. Have students identify potential unknown outcomes to illustrate "uncertainty" in decision making. (Examples: salary, what fellow workers are like, management style of supervisor.)
3. Have students identify known outcomes over which they would have no control to illustrate "risk" in decision making. (Examples: applicants will be interviewed, but will I be interviewed; someone will be selected, but will I be selected?)

ASSIGNMENT: Constructing a decision tree

Chapter objective 4 may be used as an assignment.

Objective 4: Construct a decision tree for making a professional decision:

(1) specify the problem,
(2) two alternative courses of action,
(3) two states of nature,
(5) and the expected payoff for each alternative state of nature combination.

ROLE PLAY: Responses to Decisional Conflict

Objective 3 is practiced in the following role play.

Objective 3: Describe a situation in which you experienced decisional conflict. Diagnose your response as unconflicted inertia, unconflicted change, defensive avoidance, hypervigilance, or vigilance.

Situation: Unit manager I. Candoit was assigned the responsibility of complying with a nursing care standard which staff actively resisted.

Scene: Nurse I. Candoit received memo from nursing administration requesting a progress report on the unit's compliance.

Ask for five student volunteers. Ask each student to role play response and have class identify the response Nurse I. Candoit is modeling.

1. unconflicted change

   (Nurse I. Candoit has met with staff who now see value in change and are already modifying procedures.)

2. Defensive avoidance

   (Nurse I. Candoit responds: "Oh, I forgot about that. I wonder if Sherry would work on it."

3. Unconflicted inertia

   (Nurse I. Candoit's response could include: "I am waiting to see if the standard is going to be revised when the standards committee reviews it.")

4. Hypervigilance

   (Response could include: "Sherry, this morning we were talking about the standard you are going to check on. What have you found." Three hours later, "Sherry, I have the data on the standard problem, have you had a chance to look at it yet?"

5. Vigilance

   (Return memo: "I have met with staff and shared data re. problem standard. Some are beginning to see need for change. Sherry volunteered to explore the problem with two other staff and will share their findings with me Tuesday.")

TEST QUESTIONS

KNOWLEDGE AND COMPREHENSION

True : False

T F 23.01 Decision making consists of both conscious and unconscious influences.

T F 23.02 Good management decisions are based on an understanding of all relevant causes and effects.

T F 23.03 High level management decisions stimulate low level management decisions.

T F 23.04 The purpose of a fish tail diagram is to identify the cause and effect of a problem.

T F 23.05 Use of intuition in decision making leads to biased, ineffective decisions.

Multiple Choice

23.06. Nursing management is faced with increasing difficulty in making good decisions because of:
  a. growth in information bases
  b. less competent staff
  c. reorganization of agencies
  d. all of above

23.07. The amount of psychological stress resulting from decision conflict depends on:
  a. the type of decision being made
  b. importance of decision outcome
  c. whether delegation has been used
  d. all of above

23.08. According to Jung, which of the following are psychological influences on a manager's decision making style?
  a. perception and judgment
  b. attitudes toward life
  c. attitudes toward outer world
  d. all of above

23.09. Each of the following are needed to promote good-quality decision making. In which order are they to be done?
  1. recognize need for a decision
  2. adhere to decision
  3. commit to action and implement decision
  4. determine institutional goals and priorities
  5. search for alternatives, weigh alter natives and select one
  6. identify criteria for success and identify alternative courses of action
  a. 1, 2, 3, 4, 5, 6
  b. 2, 4, 5, 6, 3, 1
  c. 3, 6, 5, 1, 2, 4
  d. 4, 1, 6, 5, 3, 2

23.10. Which step is more difficult in group decision making?
  a. problem definition
  b. problem solution options
  c. data collection, assessment
  d. decision implementation

23.11. (An) advantage(s) to "branch" decision making include:
a. based upon agency goals and priorities
b. uses problem analysis
c. small policy revisions are made until goal is achieved
d. practices scientific theory in decision making steps

23.12. When should a manager make a decision rather than use a group for decision making?
a. when time is limited
b. when need for subordinate commitment is essential
c. when the manager lacks expertise in area
d. all of above

Matching: Match the situation type to the appropriate characteristic by placing the letter in the space provided.

	Characteristic	Situation Type
____	23.13. Outcomes of a decision are unknown	a. risk
____	23.14. cannot control outcomes	b. uncertainty
____	23.15. outcomes are known	

Matching: Match the term to the definition or description by placing the letter in the space provided.

	Definition/Description	Term
____	23.16. failure to recognize possible outcomes of action	a. chameleon
____	23.17. inaccurate prediction of known action outcomes	b. decision analysis
____	23.18. decisions committing agency to long-term goals	c. error
____	23.19. decisions involving routine day-to-day operations	d. ignorance
____	23.20. strategy to frame management decision to permit variable interpretations	e. maximin
____	23.21. pessimistic approach which expects the worst when action is taken	f. mini-regret
____	23.22. approach to minimize surprise results	g. operational
____	23.23. process of breaking a complex problem into a series of simpler steps	

APPLICATION, ANALYSIS, AND/OR SYNTHESIS

Matching: Match the decision strategy used in each of the nursing actions by placing the relevant letter in the space provided.

Actions

____ 23.24. the nurse unit manager posted a holiday schedule which met the union contract, but was not ideal

____ 23.25. the nurse administrator assigned the staff nurse who identified the problem to an ad hoc committee to deal with problem

____ 23.26. the nurse manager did not act on the staff complaints of uncompleted work at the end of shift

____ 23.27. the nurse manager chooses the option that reflects the best possible action

____ 23.28. the nurse manager expects staff to respond negatively so she decides for the best approach given the anticipated negative staff response

____ 23.29. the nurse manager chooses an option which will least surprise the staff

____ 23.30. the nurse manager decides to phase in the new program in several steps over the next six months

Decision Strategies

a. do nothing

b. evolutionary

c. maximax

d. maximin

e. mini-regret

f. oppotunistic

g. satisficing

Multiple Choice

23.31. In the last week Nurse Manager Ohmy has submitted incorrectly tabulated reports, forgotten to attend a committee meeting of which she had asked to be a member, and failed to turn in the budget variance report. Nurse Manager Ohmy's behaviors are likely occurring because of:
a. information overload
b. desire to assert authority
c. disrespect of administration
d. need to control

23.32. The facility CEO opposes a decision for a new nursing service made by nursing administration because it extends services beyond the facility's mission. Which of the following most likely represents what nursing administration failed to do?
a. utilize participative management principles to promote ownership of the decision
b. practice the first step of decision making
c. establish an appropriate power base
d. all of above

23.33. Which of the following represent(s) positive actions by a nurse administrator who is experiencing information overload?
a. teach the secretary to sort and prioritize the mail and memos
b. route procedural matters to the chairperson of the Procedures Committee
c. redirect problems related to special services to persons whose job it is to address the problems
d. all of above

23.34. The unit to which Nurse Manager Smothermother has recently been assigned has experienced an unusual attrition rate of staff RNs. Upon exit interviews the resigning RNs complained "She's always telling me what to do", "She never leaves me alone." New Nurse Manager Smothermother is responding to her new role with:
a. unconflicted change
b. unconflicted inertia
c. hypervigilance
d. vigilance

23.35. Usually creative Nurse Administrator Icandoit proceeds to gather the resources to implement the proposed new nursing service which administration has rejected. The Administrator again informs Nurse Icandoit that the proposed service does not support the facility mission. Nurse Icandoit's behavior represents:
a. unconflicted inertia
b. defensive avoidance
c. hypervigilance
d. unconflicted change

23.36. The unit manager desires input from each committee member. The committee includes both very vocal and quiet members. Which of the following should the manager use?
a. brainstorming
b. nominal group process
c. fish tail diagrams
d. decision tree

Matching: Match the best management style for the situation by placing the appropriate letter in space provided.

	Situation	Best Management Style
___	23.37. The unit manager called a meeting of staff to discuss the procedural problem. Then the unit manager made the decision.	a. Autocratic I
		b. Autocratic II
		c. Consultive I
___	23.38. The nurse manager is in need of information, but the decision must be made today. She called an expert for information and made the decision.	d. Consultive II
		e. Group
___	23.39. The unit manager convenes a staff meeting to discuss the procedural problem and the group makes a decision.	
___	23.40. The informed nurse manager must make an immediate decision or there will be negative consequences.	
___	23.41. The unit manager discussed the procedural problem with each staff member and then made the decision.	

ANSWERS	TEXT REFERENCE
23.01. T	p. 418
23.02. F	p. 418, 427
23.03. T	p. 419
23.04. T	p. 429
23.05. F	p. 431
23.06. a	p. 417
23.07. b	p. 420
23.08. d	p. 426
23.09. d	p. 426, 427
23.10. a	p. 428
23.11. c	p. 428
23.12. a	p. 432
23.13. b	p. 421
23.14. a	p. 421
23.15. a	p. 421
23.16. d	p. 424
23.17. c	p. 424
23.18. h	p. 424
23.19. g	p. 422
23.20. a	p. 425
23.21. e	p. 425
23.22. f	p. 425
23.23. b	p. 431
23.24. g	p. 424
23.25. f	p. 424
23.26. a	p. 424
23.27. c	p. 424
23.28. d	p. 425
23.29. e	p. 425
23.30. b	p. 425
23.31. a	p. 419
23.32. b	p. 426
23.33. d	p. 419
23.34. c	p. 420, 421
23.35. b	p. 420
23.36. b	p. 430
23.37. d	p. 433
23.38. b	p. 433
23.39. e	p. 433
23.40. a	p. 433
23.41. c	p. 433

CHAPTER

24

Nursing Research

Research provides the foundation for professional practice. The focus on nursing research presented in chapter 24 provides a background of nursing research development, its importance, and current status. Students will be challenged by the need for better implementation of research findings in nursing practice.

KEY TERMS

C.G.E.A.N
collaborative
N.C.N.R.

OUTLINE

I. Overview
  A. Need for research
  B. History of nursing research
  C. Activities of research
    1. Generating knowledge
    2. Disseminating knowledge
    3. Using knowledge
  D. Nursing graduate level and research foci
  E. Research and practice gap
    1. Examples
    2. Causes
      a. Philosophical differences
      b. Environmental climate
  F. Steps toward adoption of research findings
    1. Knowledge
    2. Persuasion
    3. Decision
    4. Implementation
    5. Confirmation

II. Collaborative research
  A. Practice
    1. History
    2. Faculty focus
  B. Advantages
  C. Disadvantages
    1. Communications
    2. Data reliability
    3. Need to standardize procedures
    4. Resource allocations
  D. Guidelines
  E. National Center for Nursing Research
    1. List of priorities
    2. List of criteria for choosing nursing research
  F. Funding foci

1. Historical foci
2. Council on Graduate Education for Administration in Nursing

III. Encouraging research utilization by clinicians
  A. Link researchers and clinical practice setting
    1. Role of clinicians
    2. Role of researchers
    3. Dissemination of findings
  B. Promoting nurse motivation for research
    1. Use of health facility
    2. Establishment of nursing research office
    3. Nursing research relationship to nursing care quality
  C. Conduct and utilization of research in nursing project
  D. Data bases
    1. Sources
    2. Computer literacy
  E. Research staff development program
    1. Topics
    2. Resources

CLASS DISCUSSION:Topic Identification

Time: 10 minutes

PART 1 Ask students to think of the same clinical setting - a unit where they have had clinical experience. From their experiences ask them to:

Questions

1. Identify five topics of clinical research which could be applied in caring for patients.
2. Identify three topics of management research which could be applied to the unit function.

PART 2 The following activity implements objective 1.

Objective 1: List three factors that block nurses from using nursing research.

Time 10 minutes

Discussion

1. For one of the clinical research topics identified above, list three factors which might block nurses from utilizing research findings?
2. For one of the management research topics identified above, list three factors which might block utilization of research findings.

GROUP PROJECT: Clinical Nurse Researcher Position Description

Objective 3 is implemented in the following activity.

Objective 3: List four job tasks to be included in the job description of a clinical nurse researcher.

Time: 20 minutes

Identify a health care agency with which students are familiar.

Divide students in groups of five.

Tasks

1. Identify four job tasks which should in the job description of a Clinical Nurse Researcher at the identified facility.
2. Prioritize tasks and assign approximate percentage of time to be spent on each. (Tasks will not be inclusive, therefore, percentage of time should not be 100%.)

ASSIGNMENT: Research Continuing Education Program

Chapter objective 2 may be used as a written assignment or term paper.

Objective 2: Outline the contents of a continuing education program on research implementation for staff nurses.

ASSIGNMENT: Research Implementation

Assign students to find a nursing research article of interest to them, or provide three nursing research articles from which students may choose.

In writing the paper the students are to:

1. Summarize in one paragraph the study findings.
2. Discuss what would be involved in implementing the findings at the agency where students have clinical rotations. In the discussion include:
   a. How comparable is the study population to the population at the agency where the findings would be implemented.
   b. Would policy or procedural practices need to be changed. If so, which ones?
   c. Would nursing standards be impacted? If so how?
   d. Would the cost:benefit ratio be positive or negative?
   e. Would management action be required to make changes? If so, what actions would need to be taken?

TEST QUESTIONS

KNOWLEDGE AND COMPREHENSION

True : False

T F 24.01. Research based practice is part of professional practice

T F 24.02. A strong quality-management program can stimulate nursing research.

T F 24.03. The Conduct and Utilization of Research in Nursing project demonstrated that research needs to be conducted by nurse clinicians rather than nurse researchers.

Multiple Choice

24.04. Nursing research activities include:
- a. generating knowledge
- b. sharing knowledge
- c. put findings into practice
- d. all of above

24.05. Which of the following will strengthen implementation of research findings?
- a. research topics are chosen by practitioners
- b. researchers and practitioners reflect different philosophies
- c. authority for changing policy and procedures rests with practice management
- d. all of above

24.06. A collaborative research approach adds which of the following challenges?
- a. increased communication costs
- b. need to standardize data gathering procedures
- c. equitable distribution of funds
- d. all of above

APPLICATION, ANALYSIS, AND/OR SYNTHESIS

24.07. According to the text, the National Center for Nursing Research functions to:

a. focus nursing research on a few significant nursing problems
b. advocate criteria for use in setting priorities for research funding
c. recommended federal funding for nursing research for low birth weight mother:infant issues
d. all of above

24.08. Which of the following management actions would promote implementation of research findings?

a. lunches with research college faculty and shares a list of practice concerns
b. approves a staff nurse request to attend a research conference and adds at the bottom"Plan to give a short presentation of what you learn at the next nursing meeting."
c. encourages staff to participate in research activities
d. all of above

24.09. Which of the following nursing management actions will best promote staff to participate in the conduct of clinical research?

a. The manager schedules a one evening research workshop.
b. The manager works with staff to define a research problem from quality management activities.
c. The manager allocated research monies to the staff development department.
d. A BSN nurse is hired to head a nursing research department.

ANSWERS	TEXT REFERENCE
24.01. T	p. 437
24.02. T	p. 443
24.03. F	p. 443
24.04. d	p. 438
24.05. a	p. 439
24.06. d	p. 440
24.07. d	p. 441
24.08. d	p. 442
24.09 b	p. 444

CHAPTER

25

Effecting Change

The fast-paced societal, nursing, and health care delivery system changes compel the nurse manager to employ high-level change process skills. This chapter presents an arsenal of knowledge and tools with which to facilitate successful change.

OUTLINE

I. Pressures for organizational change
   A. Societal change
   B. New health care demands
   C. Research productivity
   D. Professional productivity

II. Coping with change
   A. Indicator of organizational health
   B. Six steps in coping with organizational

III. Continuity-change continuum
   A. Need to maintain balance
   B. Nurse manager's goals

IV. Variance in tolerance for change
   A. Individual differences
   B. Greater need for proactive style
   C. Need to build an organization willing to change

V. Definitions of change
   A. Change as a significant departure to status quo
   B. Change as a process

VI. Types of change
   A. Accidental or reactive
   B. Planned
   C. Levels of change
      1. First level
      2. Second level
      3. Third level
      4. Fourth level
   D. Object of change efforts
      1. Employee task behaviors
      2. Organizational processes
      3. Strategic direction
      4. Organizational culture

VII. Stages of change
   A. Unfreezing
      1. Defined
      2. Examples given
      3. Forces to unfreeze
         a. Internal forces
         b. External forces
   B. Implementing change
   C. Refreezing
   D. Using change agent

VIII. Effects of change
   A. Dynamics of change
      1. Intended change
      2. Unforeseen change
      3. Ripple effect changes
   B. Complexity shock
   C. Impact on employees

IX. Establishing a climate supportive of change
   A. Managerial behaviors
      1. Change as a norm
      2. Reward subordinates
      3. Facilitative work system
   B. Organizational self-renewal
   C. Promote teambuilding and networking
   D. Change as therapeutic process

X. Handling resistance to change
   A. Causes of resistance
      1. Requires psychological adjustment
      2. Future uncertainty
      3. Employee's investment in present
      4. Change is counter to trends
      5. Misunderstanding change process
      6. Agency's formal and informal structures
      7. Change agent characteristics or behavior
   B. Resistors
      1. Cliques
      2. Workers who oppose the change
   C. Amount of resistance
      1. Related to scope and depth of change

XI. Strategies for change
   A. Types of strategies
      1. Facilitative
      2. Informational
      3. Attitudinal
      4. Political
   B. Need for strategy
   C. Implementing strategy
      1. Through employees
      2. Through consultant
   D. Change methods
      1. Structural change
      2. Therapeutic change
      3. Unilateral authority
      4. Delegated authority
      5. Shared authority
      6. Systems approach
      7. Cyclical or "loop" strategy
      8. Authoritative approach
      9. Persuasive mode
      10. "Camel's head in the tent"
      11. Lewin's change strategy
      12. Redistribution of power
      13. Empirical-rational strategy
      14. Power-coercive
      15. Normative-re-educative

XII. Two types of plans for change
   A. Activity or performance plan
      1. Step by step of change process change
      2. Design in systems fashion
      3. Budget plan
      4. Written and signed agreement of proposed change
   B. Strategic or logistical plan
      1. Determine desirability of the change
      2. Who will be affected by change
      3. Elimination of barriers
      4. Donnely's model for selecting change strategy
      5. Inclusion of feedback loops

XIII. Tactics for change
   A. To create unrest, ask questions
   B. For diagnosis, discover discrepancy between reality and perception
   C. For introducing complex organizational change, share informally
   D. For a psychological approach, link change with personnel goals
   E. For motivation, start change with receptive persons
   F. For an objective view, use an outsider-insider pair as change agent
   G. For increased commitment, outsider performs some service that is perceived as helpful
   H. For promotion of change, present realistic expectations
   I. For confronting resistance, analyze change from adversary's viewpoint
   J. For dealing with opposition, balance assertive and oblique approaches
   K. For dealing with a clique, woo them to work for change or divide clique
   L. For presentation, stay only slightly ahead of change process
   M. For facilitating change, educate employees in problem solving and human relation skills
   N. For increasing employee support, inveigle from employee behavioral commitment to the change
   O. For unaccepting employees, practice compromise
   P. For increasing change momentum, use positive reinforcement
   Q. For organizational renewal, support middle managers
   R. For support of change targets, build a social support system

S. For discontinuous radical changes
   1. Reorient
   2. Turnaround
   3. Revitalization
   4. Transformation

XIV. The change process
   A. Steps
      1. Assessment
      2. Planning
      3. Implementation
      4. Evaluation
   B. Principles of organizational change
      1. Change represents loss to participants
      2. Match of change objective with individual personal values promotes change
      3. Involve employees in plan to promote ownership
      4. Requiring consistent demonstration of a behavior will change attitude
      5. Personal hardship increases attraction to new system
      6. Change occurs more slowly with each successive change in a series
      7. Change agent diagnoses from own perspectives
      8. Resistance increases with distance from initiator to decision maker
      9. Roles of change agent and change target should be blurred throughout change process
      10. Each innovation should provide employee learning
   C. Deterrents to change

XV. Summary

DISCUSSION IDEAS: Promoting change

Situation: Use the situation of the Problem ADON in the GROUP ACTIVITY for Chapter 21 in this *Manual* as a background.

I. Levels of change

The following questions pertain to chapter objective 2: "Give an example of one first-level, one second-level, one third-level, and one fourth-level change in your health agency and speculate about the probable cause and effect(s) of each."

Administration has decided that the ADON is blocking progressive changes in nursing. The ADON must change her behaviors, be encouraged to resign, or be placed in a different position.

1. To promote a change in ADON behaviors, state actions administration could implement to achieve:
   - first-level change
   - second-level change
   - third-level change
   - fourth-level change.
2. Which level of change must be achieved prior to the ADON's ability to practice participative management?

II. Stages of change

The next questions pertain to chapter objective 3: "Describe one action by a manger to facilitate each of the following stages of a change in your nursing department: a. unfreezing, b moving, c. refreezing."

The ADON must make a change to which the nursing union membership is opposed. Utilize Chapter 25 of the text as a reference in answering the following questions.

1. How might the ADON "woo" the union membership? What actions can the ADON try?
2. If the ADON is unable to "woo" the union membership, what actions could the ADON take to dilute the resistance of the union membership?

GROUP PROJECT: Strategic and Activity planning

The activities for this project demonstrate the desired learning of chapter objective 4: "Outline a four to five step strategic plan and a four to five step activity plan for a functional change in your nursing organization.

Time: The project is best conducted as an outside assignment or divided into two class periods: one for strategic planning and one for activity planning.

Situation: Utilize the Topseyturvey Hospital's Outpatient Surgery and Diagnostic Center situation presented in the Group Activity for Chapter 22 of this *Manual* as background.

However, Nurse Naivette will be wiser in her approach to initiating change. She will first outline a strategic plan and an activity plan for setting up all aspects of the new Outpatient Surgery and Diagnostic Center.

Assignment

1. You are wise Nurse Naivette. Outline a strategic plan to be followed.
2. Outline an activity plan.

TEST QUESTIONS

KNOWLEDGE AND COMPREHENSION

True : False

T F 25.01. The nurse manager is practicing activity planning when she analyzes whether or not to attempt change.

T F 25.02. A statement of the future reality resulting from a change is part of strategic planning.

T F 25.03. A key criteria for judging organizational health is the organization's ability to cope with change.

T F 25.04. An employee's resistance to change is proportional to her or his emotional investment in status quo.

APPLICATION, ANALYSIS, AND/OR SYNTHESIS

Matching: Match the stage of change process represented by the managerial behaviors by placing the appropriate letter in the space provided.

Managerial Behaviors

____ 25.05. The positive effects of the new system are shared with the involved staff

____ 25.06. Identify the employee dissatisfiers and relate a positive effect on the dissatisfiers by the proposed change

____ 25.07. The nurses believe that care continuity is necessary for quality care and therefore are receptive to implementing primary nursing

____ 25.08. The nurse manager shares the deficiencies cited by the accreditation team

Stage of Change Process

a. unfreezing

b. moving

c. refreezing

Multiple Choice

25.09. The Podville Hospital nursing department recognizes the need to adjust nursing services to better serve the aging population of their community and changes their nursing philosophy orientation from a biological systems model to a developmental model. This action demonstrates:
a. responsiveness to a societal change
b. following a nursing "fad"
c. unmerited change
d. the implementation step of change

25.10. What level(s) of change will occur in the staff nurses through the implementation of a developmental model in their philosophy in the situation used in the above question?
a. first-level change and second-level change
b. third-level change
c. fourth-level change
d. a and b
e. a, b, and c

25.11. The nursing administrator practices an autocratic style of leadership. To help the nursing administrator move into a more participative leadership style the CEO forwards articles about participative leadership to the nursing administrator. The nursing administrator realizes the leadership style s/he practices is autocratic and stagnates subordinate growth. What level of change is represented in this situation?
a. first-level
b. second-level
c. third-level
d. fourth level

25.12. Nurse unit managers propose being responsible for staffing their respective units because of problems arising out of centralized staffing. The organization practices bureaucratic decision making, and the nurse administrator values control. What is the likelihood of the proposed change occurring?
a. highly likely
b. probable
c. possible with much effort
d. unlikely

25.13. Staff nurse Iwanit would like for her nursing unit to add a new nursing service. The nursing unit is currently understaffed and using costly pool nurses. She begins outlining strategic and activity plans for the new nursing service. What is the likelihood of Nurse Iwanit being able to move this change forward?
a. highly likely
b. probable
c. possible with much effort
d. unlikely

25.14. Which of the following nurse administrator action will facilitate organizational change?
a. One day a week is designated as a problem solving and "futures" day for unit managers.
b. A recognition, incentive program was established to reward staff members who contribute to problem solving efforts.
c. The administrator worked with unit managers to redesign unit manager job descriptions to include greater autonomy.
d. all of above

Matching: Match the change strategy used in each of the situations by placing the appropriate letter in the space provided.

Situations

____ 25.15. The unit manager helped staff to develop a proposal for a policy change that staff wanted.

____ 25.16. The unit manager shared quality improvement findings to staff. Staff were surprised at the findings.

____ 25.17. The nurse administrator wisely waited until staff saw a need for the change.

____ 25.18. Two-thirds of staff development is designated for management oriented learning activities for next budget period.

____ 25.19. Administration hired a consultant management educator to grow unit managers in management skills.

____ 25.20. The unit manager asked staff to try out the new procedure for six weeks.

Change Strategies

a. attitudinal

b. facilitative

c. informational

d. loop

e. persuasive

f. political

ANSWERS	TEXT REFERENCE
25.01. F	p. 462, 463
25.02. F	p. 463
25.03. T	p. 450
25.04. T	p. 457
25.05. c	p. 453, 454
25.06. a	p. 453, 454
25.07. b	p. 453, 454
25.08. a	p. 453, 454
25.09. a	p. 448, 449
25.10. d	p. 451, 452
25.11. a	p. 451
25.12. d	p. 469
25.13. d	p. 455, 456
25.14. d	p. 455, 456
25.15. b	p. 458
25.16. c	p. 459
25.17. a	p. 458
25.18. f	p. 458, 459
25.19. d	p. 459, 460
25.20. e	p. 460

CHAPTER

26

Managing Conflict

The management of conflicts requires high cognitive and interpersonal skills by the manager. In this chapter the student considers a wide range of conflict causes and is challenged to identify basic underlying issues, separating them from substituted or manufactured issues. The steps, phases, and consequences of conflict are considered as are intervention modes. The role playing activity will provide students an opportunity of learning about these various aspects of managing conflict.

KEY TERMS

compromise
concession
conflict
confrontation
effective expression
empathic responding
mediator

OUTLINE

I. Introduction
   A. Definition
   B. Conflict as a constructive force

II. Causes of conflict
   A. Frustration of basic needs
   B. Change
   C. Professional interdependence
   D. Psychological closeness
   E. Differing perceptions
   F. Role ambiguity, disagreement
   G. Highly differentiated positions
   H. Role changes
   I. Role ambiguity
   J. Substantive causes
   K. Emotional causes
   L. The unknown
   M. Unworkable organization structure
   N. Power disequilibrium

III. Effects of conflict
   A. Positive
      1. Clears air
      2. Prevents groupthink
      3. Provides intellectual stimulation
      4. Promotes problem solving
      5. Facilitates personal maturation
   B. Negative
      1. Anxiety
      2. Defensiveness
      3. Flee workplace

IV. Nature of conflict
   A. Stages of conflict
      1. Latent hostility

2. Open hostility
3. Withdrawal from conflict
4. Cyclical

B. Persistence of conflict
1. Conflict changes
2. Disputants change

C. Direct or indirect conflict

D. Escalation of conflict
1. Commitment to position increases
2. Additional issues are added
3. Antagonism carries from issue to individuals
4. Conflict attracts additional combatants
5. De-escalation of conflict does not equal resolution

E. Unfavorable termination of conflict

F. Use of scape-goating

V. Analysis of conflict
A. Overview
B. Roles in conflict situations
1. Aggressor
2. Victim
3. Investigator
4. Cliques
C. Issues underlying conflict
1. Identify principal issue
2. Discriminate from substitute issue
3. Manufacturing of issues
D. Types of conflict
1. Direct examples
2. Indirect examples
3. Physician:nurse
E. Phases of conflict development
1. Differentiation
2. Integration
3. Conflict transformation
a. Splitting
b. Projection
c. Triangulation
F. Severity of conflict
G. Consequences of conflict
1. Low and moderate stress increases problem-solving abilities
2. High stress levels decrease quality of intellectual processes
3. Chronic stress

VI. Intervention in conflict
A. Intervention
1. Need
2. Motives
3. Timing
a. Readiness of disputants
b. Escalate conflict to precipitate need
4. Site
5. Conduct
6. Plan
7. Approaches
a. Eliminate underlying cause
b. Separate disputants
c. Apply positional authority
8. Manager's style
a. High relationship
b. High task
c. High relationship and high task
d. Social style
B. Responsibilities of the mediator
1. Responsibilities
a. Determine motivation for conflict and for negotiation
b. Equalize situational power
c. Synchronize disputants
d. Clarify claims
2. Promote active listening by disputants
3. Identify key themes
4. Encourage feedback
5. Facilitate expression
a. Effective expression
b. Empathic responding
6. Prepare disputants
7. Methods to resolve conflict
a. Phillip's and Cheston's four methods
b. Blake and Mouton's two methods
c. Jendt's multiple issue conflict
C. Confrontation
1. Description
2. Use
3. Stages

VII. Outcomes of intervention
A. No resolution
B. Concession
C. Compromise
D. Integrated solution
E. Follow-up on agreed actions
F. Separate parties when conflict is unresolvable

VIII. Summary

CLASS ACTIVITY: Conflict resolution analysis; role play

The following activities address chapter objectives 1, 2, and 4.

Time: 1 - 2 class periods

Ask two students to role play the situation before the class.

Situation

Scene I.: After searching for three months, Nurse Iamhere was hired for ICU. She has extensive ICU experience. Nurse Iamhere refused to take her turn to float out of the unit when the census was down because she was hired for ICU and it is ICU nursing she wants to do. A more senior ICU nurse, Ms. Oletimer was floated out of the unit instead.

Scene II.: Since that time Nurse Oletimer frequently complains about inconsequential things that Nurse Iamhere has done. Nurse morale is deteriorating on the unit and patient care is suffering.

Scene III.: Nurse Iamhere is talking about taking a position at another facility because people are so hard to get along with here.

Objective 2: Analyze a conflict between yourself and a coworker, and identify substantive and emotional causes for the conflict.

Questions

1. What are the substantive issues:
   - from Nurse Iamhere's viewpoint?
   - from Nurse Oletimer's viewpoint?
2. What are the emotional issues:
   - from Nurse Iamhere's viewpoint?
   - from Nurse Oletimer's viewpoint?
3. At what point is intervention needed?

Objective 1: Identify aspects of your professional role that predispose to conflict with nurse administrator or physicians.

Questions

1. Expectancy discrepancies are a frequent cause of conflict. Identify expectancy discrepancies between

   a. Nurse Iamhere and administration.

   b. Nurse Iamhere and Nurse Oletimer.

Objective 4: Analyze an ongoing conflict in your agency, and identify the original conflict issue and secondary issues that were raised as the dispute escalated.

Questions

1. What are the basic substantive issue and the secondary issues involved from the viewpoint of each nurse?
2. What are the basic emotional issue and the secondary emotional issues involved from the viewpoint of each nurse?
3. If you were the mediator, *what* would you recommend and *how* would you accomplish the recommendation?

Situation

Choose a student to role play the nurse manager.

The nurse manager is to use an authoritative resolution to the conflict.

Question

Ask Nurse Iamhere and Nurse Oletimer each how they react to the resolution of the conflict.

Situation continued

The nurse manager calls the two together to express their differences and to facilitate their arriving at their own solution.

Question

Elicit from the class how the nurse manager is to play the role. Have the class give examples of what the nurse manager is to say and do.

ROLES ARE PLAYED OUT

1. What role did each of the disputants play in the conflict resolution?
2. Ask role players how they each feel regarding the conflict resolution.
3. Have class identify examples of mediating behaviors, facilitating clarification, and feedback.

(Faculty: Because of basic managerial substantive issues, the conflict will not be totally resolved by placing ownership on the disputants.)

Guide students to identify managerial issues and suggest solutions. (Objective 4)

Situation continued

The nurse manager plans to implement the class's suggested solutions and thus take part ownership for the conflict. The nurse manager then calls Nurse Iamhere and Nurse Oletimer in to identify the issues and together agree upon resolutions.

Questions

1. What role did each of the disputants play this time?
2. Ask role players how they each feel regarding the conflict resolution.
3. Have class again identify examples of mediating behaviors.

ASSIGNMENT: Role predisposition to conflict

Chapter objective 1 can be used as a short (four page) assignment for RN students.

Objective 1: Identify aspects of your professional role that predispose to conflict with nurse administrators or physicians.

Assignment

1. In one paragraph describe the situation out of which role conflict arises. Include a description of the conflict. (1 page)
2. What are the conflict issues which revolve around role issues? (1 page)
3. Should the conflict continue, what are the likely effects? (1 page)
4. What intervention(s) would you suggest to resolve the conflict? (1 page)

TEST QUESTIONS

KNOWLEDGE AND COMPREHENSION

True : False

T F 26.01. Conflict has a unifying effect on a work force.

T F 26.02. In a close working relationship conflict is less likely to occur.

T F 26.03. Conflict is dynamic and cyclical.

T F 26.04. Identification of a scapegoat by a group will be a disintegrating force.

T F 26.05. The greatest difficulty in analyzing conflict development is to decide if integration is occurring.

T F 26.06. Conflicts become expressed at locations far removed from origin.

T F 26.07. A moderate level of conflict stimulates creative thinking.

Multiple Choice

26.08. Substantive causes of conflict include:
a. disagreements over policies or procedures
b. competition for scarce resources
c. pressure for cost containment
d. all of above

26.09. Advantages of conflict include:
a. foster problem solving
b. provides impetus for personal growth
c. prevents stagnation
d. all of above

26.10. Which of the following occur(s) when conflict persists?
a. nature of hostilities/problem changes
b. the conflict will resolve itself given time
c. involved individuals will compromise and resolve issue
d. all of above

26.11. To intervene successfully the nurse manager must _?_ and _?_.
a. analyze conflict carefully
b. diagnose conflict accurately
c. devise solution to the conflict
d. implement solution

26.12. In any conflict situation the manager must identify persons in which roles?
a. leader, scapegoat, followers
b. compromiser(s), withdrawn person(s), hostile person(s)
c. aggressor, victim, instigator
d. originator, person providing on-going fuel to conflict, persons effected by conflict

26.13. Emotional causes of conflict include:
a. distrust, fear
b. interpersonal conflict
c. power disequilibrium
d. all of above

APPLICATION, ANALYSIS, AND/OR SYNTHESIS

Multiple Choice

26.14. The primary nurse enjoys the autonomy of her nursing practice. A new head nurse is accustomed to managing a unit that practices functional nursing and tells the primary nurse that she is responsible for all the heparin locks. The primary nurse responds negatively. This is an example of conflict arising out of:

a. incongruities between role definition
b. indirect conflict
c. latent conflict
d. psychological closeness

26.15. Nurse Wiseone correctly diagnosed problems with which the group did not want to deal. The group forced Nurse Wiseone to resign. Nurse Wiseone was the:

a. aggressor
b. instigator
c. scapegoat
d. leader

26.16. Nurse Noway made up an excuse to explain why she did not want to work with Nurse Purrfect. The reason for manufacturing an excuse was likely that:

a. Nurse Noway was fearful of being seen negatively if the real reason was stated.
b. Nurse Noway does not know the basic underlying cause of the conflict.
c. Nurse Purrfect would not do her share of the work.
d. Role reversal is occurring.

26.17. Which of the following is/are facilitating behavior(s) to be practiced in the role of the mediator?

a. meet with the disadvantaged party and help the party prepare for the conference
b. encourage frequent feedback
c. promote effective expression
d. all of above

ANSWERS	TEXT REFERENCE
26.01. T	p. 472
26.02. F	p. 473
26.03. T	p. 475
26.04. F	p. 477
26.05. F	p. 479
26.06. T	p. 479
26.07. T	p. 480
26.08. d	p. 473, 474
26.09. d	p. 475
26.10. a	p. 476
26.11. a and b	p. 477
26.12. c	p. 477
26.13. a	p. 480
26.14. a	p. 474, 475, 476
26.15. c	p. 477
26.16. a	p. 478
26.17. d	p. 483, 484

CHAPTER

27

Computer Information Systems

The wise nursing manager will become familiar with computers and what computers can do for nursing practice, management, and patient care. The nurse manager wants to choose computer systems which aid in controlling the various nursing functions and to avoid computer systems which are served by nursing and are in themselves the controllers. The content of the chapter presents a comfortably understandable and pragmatic overview of computer information systems.

OUTLINE

I. Overview
    A. Need for unified system
    B. Purpose of unified system
    C. Role of computers

II. Systems theory
    A. A model for computer use
    B. Identification of elements
    C. Integration of parts

III. Computer system
    A. Applications
        1. Management
        2. Nursing practice
        3. Patient records
            a. Content examples
            b. Bedside terminal advantages
    B. System types
        1. Nursing information systems
            a. Patient oriented information
            b. Quality monitoring
        2. Management information system
            a. Purpose
            b. Software tools
            c. Uses
        3. Hospital information system
    C. Process of computerizing information systems
        1. Planning committee
            a. Nurse role
            b. Review manual systems
            c. Tasks
        2. Reviewing software
        3. Use of flowcharts
            a. Role
            b. Description
            c. Construction

IV. Disadvantages of computerized information systems
    A. Confidentiality
    B. Increased work pace
    C. Increased expectancies
    D. Increasing impersonality of interactions
    E. Segmentation of work force

V. Artificial intelligence applications
   A. Definitions
      1. Nursing information
      2. Data
      3. Information
      4. Knowledge
      5. Decision making system
         a. Automated
         b. Decision support systems
   B. Expert systems
      1. Parts
         a. Knowledge base
         b. Inference engine
         c. Knowledge interface
            (1). Temporal string
            (2). Heuristic rules
               (a). Forward chaining
               (b). Backward chaining
            (3). spatial image
      2. Examples
         a. Non-medical
         b. Florence (nursing)
            (1). Content
            (2). Use process
         c. Medical examples
            (1). Psychiatric
            (2). Nutritional
            (3). Sarah
            (4). Home-bound monitoring
         d. Maintenance management example
   C. Computer simulations for nursing
      1. Description
      2. Use
      3. Examples
   D. Computer assisted instruction (CAI)
      1. Linear instruction programs
      2. Branching instruction programs
      3. Intelligent computer assisted instruction
         a. Description
         b. Use
   E. System development
      1. Extracting knowledge
         a. Learning through instruction, observation
         b. Practicing to proficiency
         c. Overpractice to automatic
      2. Development of rules of thumb
      3. Process development example
      4. "Shell" program
VI. Summary

CLASS DISCUSSION IDEAS: Use of computers to serve nursing

Chapter objectives 1, and 2 can provide good discussion material.

Objective 1: Describe three nursing activities that can be facilitated through computerization.

Questions

1. How are computers now being used to support nursing practice in the facility with which you are familiar?
2. What are additional functions that could be done by computers to better serve nursing practice?

Objective 2: List three nursing management functions that can be facilitated through computerization.

Questions

1. How is nursing management using computers in the facility with which you are familiar?
2. What are additional functions that could be done by computers to better serve nursing management?

   (Questions 3 and 4 are best used for RN managers.)

3. Is nurse management experiencing information overload because of computer-generated information?
4. How might the computer-generated information be presented and/or routed to better serve nursing management?

GROUP PROJECT: Planning for a computerized quality improvement system

The project will implement the purpose of chapter objective 3: "Indicate three types of information that a vice-president of nursing should give a vendor from whom she wishes to purchase an automated nursing information system.
Time: 30 minutes for questions 1 and 2.
30 minutes for question 3.

Situation

Each group is to function as an Ad Hoc Committee which is charged with the task of choosing software for Podville Hospital's Quality Assurance program. The group is meeting in preparation for a meeting with vendors, and review of products.

Activities

1. The text suggests information the vendor will want to know. Create this information.

2. The text suggests information that you will want to know. Write the questions you will ask of the vendor.

3. The text further suggests that a model for decision making be followed in scheduling implementation of a computer system. Outline the steps which need to be taken from inception of the idea to implementation of a quality information computer system.

TEST QUESTIONS

KNOWLEDGE AND COMPREHENSION

True : False

T F 27.01. A purpose of an integrated health information system is to provide timely distribution of patient data.

T F 27.02. When planning for a computerized nursing information system, software should be chosen before hardware.

T F 27.03. A flow chart is used to record vitals on a bedside computer.

Matching: Match the focus of the computer system to the example of information the computer system generates by placing the relevant letter in the space provided.

Information Use

____ 27.04. produces information for executives, middle managers, and service employees to facilitate decision making

____ 27.05. patient classification system

____ 27.06. timely management of patient-related information to ensure coordinated interventions

____ 27.07. monitoring of patient physiological functions

____ 27.08. scheduling, quality assurance, nursing budget

____ 27.09. "in-basket" program

Computer System Focus

a. HIS

b. MIS

c. nursing management

d. nursing practice

e. simulation

Multiple Choice

27.10. Which of the following would be characteristic of bedside computer use?
  a. increased documentation accuracy
  b. ready acceptance by physicians
  c. increased graphing
  d. all of above

27.11. *Disadvantage(s)* of computer information systems include:
  a. increased expectations
  b. confidentiality problems
  c. increasing impersonality
  d. all of above

27.12. Which of the following describe(s) the Florence system?
  a. identifies nursing diagnoses
  b. is a case based nursing expert system
  c. is both a staff development and a job guide tool
  d. all of above

27.13. Expert computer systems now exist for:
  a. nutritional problems
  b. monitoring home-bound patients
  c. psychiatric disorders
  d. all of above

APPLICATION, ANALYSIS, AND/OR SYNTHESIS

Multiple Choice

27.14. The nursing administrator is scheduled to meet with a software vendor about a NIS. What information will she gather prior to the meeting?
  a. nursing department goals for the system
  b. size and character of the nursing department
  c. the number and sophistication of anticipated users
  d. all of above

27.15. The statement "14 of the 23 possible MI patients were discharged within 5 days" is an example of:
  a. expert information
  b. data
  c. knowledge
  d. all of above

27.16. The statement "the quality information study demonstrated the relationship between PCA use and post operative patient care satisfaction" is an example of:
  a. expert information
  b. data
  c. knowledge
  d. all of above

27.17. Which of the following systems would be useful to a nurse practitioner in a rural setting?
  a. HIS
  b. Florence
  c. decision sup port
  d. all of above

ANSWERS	TEXT REFERENCE
27.01. T	p. 491, 492
27.02. T	p. 496
27.03. F	p. 497
27.04. b	p. 494
27.05. c	p. 494
27.06. a	p. 495
27.07. d	p. 494
27.08. c	p. 494
27.09. e	p. 504
27.10. a	p. 493
27.11. d	p. 497, 499
27.12. d	p. 501, 502
27.13. d	p. 502, 503
27.14. d	p. 496
27.15. b	p. 499
27.16. c	p. 499
27.17. c	p. 499

CHAPTER

28

Quality Improvement

Quality improvement activities have evolved from limited structure and process activities, and strong use of retrospective chart audits to multidisciplinary continuous quality improvement activities based upon critical indicators. Nursing is challenged to maintain focus on ongoing improvement of concurrent patient care. The several quality improvement assignments presented in this chapter may be used to introduce and/or update students in current quality improvement practices.

KEY TERMS

benchmarking
concurrent audits
critical indicators
norm
outcome
peer review
P.E.P.
process
rate based indicator
reliability
retrospective audits
sentinel event indicator
structure
validity

OUTLINE

I. Introduction
  A. Need for quality improvement
  B. Historical quality improvement activities
II. Demand for quality improvement
  A. Historical
  B. Professional
    1. JCAHO
    2. American Nurses' Association (ANA)
III. Joint Commission's quality improvement program
  A. A condition for accreditation
  B. Standards
    1. Multidisciplinary focus
    2. Hospital examples
    3. Long term care examples
  C. Critical indicators
  D. Corrective action
  E. PEP auditing
IV. ANA quality improvement program
  A. Standards development
    1. Rose out of 1970s
    2. Process oriented
    3. Examples
  B. Clinical nursing standards
    1. Care

2. Professional performance

V. Definitions
   A. Philosophy
   B. Accountability
   C. Nursing care outcome
   D. Criterion
   E. Standard
   F. Norm
   G. Objective
   H. Critical clinical indicator
   I. Measurement
   J. Feedback
   K. Quality health care
   L. Quality assurance
   M. Continuous quality improvement
   N. Effectiveness
   O. Efficiency
   P. Peer
   P. Nursing peer review

VI. Approaches to quality improvement
   A. Framework
      1. Structure
      2. Process
         a. Nursing process
         b. Subsystems to achieve nursing process
      3. Outcomes
   B. Historical evolution of frameworks

VII. Principles underlying quality improvements efforts
   A. All health care professionals should collaborate
   B. Coordination is needed
   C. Resource expenditure for quality improvement needs to be appropriate
   D. Monitor critical performance factors
   E. Key to ensuring quality care is accurate evaluation of care
   F. Ability to achieve objectives rests on entire nursing process
   G. Evaluation of care will not by itself improve practice
   H. Peer pressure can provide impetus for needed change
   I. Changes at unit level may require changes in formal organizational structure
   J. Analysis of quality improvement data must be performed by a decision maker

VIII. Implementing a quality improvement program
   A. Process overview
   B. Quality improvement task force
      1. Task force
         a. Representation
         b. Member preparation
      2. Concurrence on beliefs and values re. quality improvement
      3. Topics
         a. Selecting
         b. Prioritizing

IX. Quality improvement methods
   A. Ongoing process
   B. Purpose
      1. To measure
      2. To improve
   C. Identifying clinical indicators of quality care
      1. Description of critical clinical indicator
      2. Types
         a. Structure
         b. Process
         c. Outcome
         d. Sentinel
         e. Rate
      3. Development guidelines
   D. Reliability and validity of measuring tools
      1. Reliability
         a. Definition
         b. Methods
      2. Validity
         a. Definition
         b. High and low validity examples
   E. Examples of quality improvement criteria
      1. Format
      2. Use of expert knowledge
      3. Use of nursing process
      4. Use of outcome criteria
   F. Testing quality improvement criteria
   G. Preparation of the measurement tool
      1. Guiding format
         a. Use of ANA standards
         b. Use of generic nursing care plans
         c. Use of nursing process and its subsystems
      2. Constructing tool
         a. User considerations
         b. Acceptable standards

XI. Total quality management
   A. Background
   B. Steps for implementation

- C. Continuous process
  1. Responsibility
  2. Improvement focus
  3. Systems viewpoint
- D. Benchmarking
- E. Training and motivating nursing staff
  1. Critical indicators, criteria
  2. Positive and negative motivation foci
     a. Investment in status quo
     b. Educational perspective
     c. Avoidance of guilt
     d. Promotion through linkage with job satisfiers
     e. Quality improvement as a learning activity
- F. Types of patient care audits
  1. Topical examples
  2. Methodological examples
     a. Concurrent
     b. Retrospective
- G. Performing the audit
  1. Determine sample size
  2. Establish who is to perform reviews
  3. Analysis of medical record data
     a. Identify charts showing variation from criteria
     b. Examples of nursing audit, need identification, and corrective action
     c. Need for feedback to those performing audited criteria

XII. Peer review
- A. Definition
- B. Characteristics
  1. Development of performance evaluation criteria
     a. Job description
     b. ANA practice standards
  2. Development of performance appraisal tool
  3. Determine who is to do evaluation
     a. Identify who is to appraise each aspect
     b. Use of self-appraisal
  4. Activities

XIII. Quality circles
- A. History
- B. Giving feedback to staff
  1. Distribution plan
  2. Choosing reportable data
  3. Reinforce staff through positive feedback
  4. Mode for sharing
  5. Distribute feedback at all levels
- C. Remedying deficiencies
  1. Staff development and educational activities
  2. Counseling or job enrichment
  3. Established practices to minimize sensory overload
  4. Discipline

XIV. Problems associated with quality improvement efforts
- A. Loss of focus on improving nursing care
- B. Lack of accurate behavioral measurement
- C. Lack of an established, known superior approach
- D. Relationships to other variables
- E. Inability to measure all variables
- F. Difficulty in defining nursing influence
- G. Documentation deficiencies
- H. Lack of universality of assessment tools

XV. Summary

GROUP PROJECT: Structure, process, outcome criterion

Chapter objective 1 may be used as an activity: "Write one structure criterion, one process criterion, and one outcome criterion to evaluate nursing care quality for patients with a specific medical or nursing diagnosis."

Time: 15- 20 minutes plus discussion time

Divide the class into three or more groups.
One group is to be assigned the task of writing a structure criterion.
One group is to be assigned the task of writing a process criterion.
One group is to be assigned the task of writing an outcome criterion.

Reconvene class. Have each group present their criterion and state rationale for why it is a structure, or process, or outcome criterion.

GROUP ASSIGNMENT: Quality Improvement Survey

Objectives 1 and 3 will be met through the assignment and the focus of objective 4 will be addressed.

Objective 1: Write one structure criterion, one process criterion, and one outcome criterion to evaluate nursing care quality for patients with a specific medical or nursing diagnosis

Objective 3: Identify three topics that would be suitable for ongoing quality monitoring in you nursing unit, and explain reasons for selecting each.

Objective 4: Perform a concurrent process audit of a selected nursing procedure on your nursing unit.

The assignment could also be used as a term paper.

Preparation: Reproduce Figures 28.1 and 28.2 (at the back of this *Manual*) for each student.

Have students group themselves into groups of three.

Assignment

1. Select one of group to interview a nurse unit manager. Share assignment with the manager. Complete Figures 28.1 and Figures 28.2 during the interview. If time is limited, explain the assignment and arrange to pick up completed survey at a designated time. State that you will share your results when the assignment is finished.

2. Group activities

   a. Review survey

   b. Choose the concern in each category which merits the most immediate attention.

c. Write one critical indicator to use in on-going quality improvement activity to address each of the concerns identified in "b" above.

3. Report content

   a. Attach surveys to paper.

   b. State each concern chosen under 2b above giving rationale for choice.

   c. State critical indicator to be used for each identified concern.

4. Share report with nurse manager

GROUP ASSIGNMENT:

ASSIGNMENT: PREPARING FOR AN AUDIT.

The activity will incorporate chapter objectives 1, 2, and 4.

Objective 1: Write one structure criterion, one process criterion, and one outcome criterion to evaluate nursing care quality for patients with a specific medical or nursing diagnosis.

Objective 2: Explain why training nursing personnel to use a quality-monitoring tool increases the reliability of the tool.

Objective 4: Perform a concurrent process audit of a selected nursing procedure on your nursing unit.

Situation

You are the nurse unit manager of Podville Hospital's Over 70s unit. (See Chapter 13 of this *Manual* for background regarding the Over 70s unit.) You are responsible for performing a patient care audit focusing on outcomes.

Activities: In three to five typed pages

1. Identify a suitable topic for a patient care outcome audit.
2. Identify critical indicators.
3. Determine the way in which the audit will be conducted.
4. List the steps to be taken to properly prepare and conduct the audit.

CLINICAL ASSIGNMENT: Concurrent process audit

Chapter objective 4 may be used as a clinical assignment: "Perform a concurrent process audit of a selected nursing procedure on your own nursing unit."

TEST QUESTIONS

KNOWLEDGE AND COMPREHENSION

True : False

T F 28.01. Nurses are unilaterally responsible for quality assurance.

T F 28.02. To promote effectiveness of quality improvement efforts the collection and analysis of data must be made by one with decision making authority.

T F 28.03. Continuing quality improvement is part of the professional role of nurses.

T F 28.04. Nursing has accumulated a repertoire of reliable outcome criteria.

T F 28.05. Over enthusiastic support of a unit manager for quality improvement activities may alienate uncommitted staff.

T F 28.06. Negative quality improvement findings are best conveyed in writing.

T F 28.07. Nursing documentation is a major problem when performing retrospective chart audits.

Multiple Choice

28.08. The role of JCAHO in quality improvement includes:
- a. recommended standards
- b. recommended critical indicators
- c. audit methods
- d. all of above

28.09. JCAHO 1992 recommendations for long term care included focus on:
- a. compartmentalizing quality improvement activities in accordance with organizational structure
- b. work groups
- c. managerial issues
- d. all of above

28.10. ANA's 1991 guide to nursing standards recognizes standards:
- a. for identifying critical indicators
- b. establishing expert criteria
- c. of care and of professional performance
- d. all of above

28.11. Quality improvement staff education should include:
- a. purpose
- b. beliefs and values
- c. methods
- d. all of above

28.12. Which of the following employees will be involved in total, continuous quality management?
- a. staff nurses
- b. nurses on other units
- c. patients
- d. all of above

28.13. Which of the following is best described as a group of employees who meet to solve work related problems, and recommend solutions to management?
- a. union
- b. quality circle
- c. Pareto group
- d. peer evaluation group

APPLICATION, ANALYSIS, AND/OR SYNTHESIS

MATCHING: Match the focus to the quality improvement activity by placing the relevant letter in the space provided.

Quality Improvement Activity

____ 28.14. The chart audit was to determine to what extent evaluation of care was documented.

____ 28.15. The nurse unit managers are to complete a budget variance analysis.

____ 28.16. The patient survey questionnaire asked if the patient would recommend the services to friends and/or relatives.

____ 28.17. Incontinent patients for whom the new brand of absorbent pads was used had fewer skin breaks than the group for whom the old brand of absorbent pads was used.

____ 28.18. The audit focused on whether a comprehensive intake patient assessment was completed.

____ 28.19. The units were instructed to inventory all equipment with working parts to ensure its functioning.

____ 28.20. The number of in patient days for a given DRG was reduced when primary nursing care was implemented.

Focus

a. outcome

b. process

c. structure

MATCHING: Match the term to the illustrative example by placing the appropriate letter in the space provided.

	Illustrative Example	Term
___	28.21. nine of ten patients bedridden for eight days were free of pressure sores	a. criterion
		b. critical clinical indicator
___	28.22. amount and type of nursing education	c. evaluation
		d. norm
___	28.23. all nursing managers will have a minimum of a bachelors degree within one year	e. nursing care outcome
		f. peer review
___	28.24. an individualized care plan was completed within eight hours of admission for 60% of the patients	g. standard
___	28.25. postoperative hemorrhage, postoperative pneumonia, urinary tract infection	
___	28.26. after reviewing quality improvement data the nurse manager was pleased to identify the occurrence of fewer patient falls	
___	28.27. Unit I nurses used preestablished standards to audit specified Unit II nursing care activities	

Multiple Choice

28.28. The patient care audit followed a certain treatment procedure to determine patient outcomes related to the treatment. This audit is attempting to measure:

a. the effectiveness of the nursing intervention.
b. the efficiency of the nursing intervention.
c. the degree to which criteria are being achieved.
d. all of above.

28.29. Each nurse unit manager is to conduct an audit on her unit. A training session for the nurse unit managers included the use of the audit criteria, a practice session of applying the criteria, and reinstruction where large differences existed. The purpose of the training session is to:

a. practice peer review
b. increase the validity of the audit
c. increase the reliability of the audit
d. all of above

28.30. Which quality improvement method would provide the best opportunity of improving nursing interventions of a current patient?
   a. retrospective chart audit
   b. structure monitoring
   c. ongoing outcome monitoring
   d. patient satisfaction survey

ANSWERS	TEXT REFERENCE
28.01. F	p. 518
28.02. T	p. 518
28.03. T	p. 518
28.04. F	p. 522
28.05. T	p. 525
28.06. F	p. 530
28.07. T	p. 532
28.08. a	p. 512, 513
28.09. C	p. 512, 513
28.10. c	p. 514
28.11. d	p. 519
28.12. d	p. 524
28.13. d	p. 502, 503
28.14. b	p. 517
28.15. c	p. 517
28.16. c	p. 517
28.17. a	p. 517
28.18. b	p. 517
28.19. c	p. 517
28.20. a	p. 520
28.21. e	p. 515
28.22. a	p. 515
28.23. g	p. 515
28.24. d	p. 515
28.25. b	p. 515, 520
28.26. c	p. 516
28.27. f	p. 516
28.28. a	p. 516
28.29. c	p. 521, 524
28.30. c	p. 519

CHAPTER

29

Performance Appraisal

A primary goal of performance appraisal is to improve employee performance. The principles of evaluation and the practical information on tools and conduct of evaluation processes presented in the text will serve as a handy reference to the nurse manager who wants to promote positive employee growth. Through the role playing activity BSN students will experience both difficulties and positive approaches of useful performance appraisal.

KEY TERMS

BARS
bias
central tendency error
forced choice
free response
graphic rating scale
halo effect
horns effect
MBO
objectivity
ranking tool
"trigger" words

OUTLINE

I. Overview
   A. Description of employee performance
   B. Role of performance appraisals
      1. Controlling mechanism
      2. Evaluation of employees
      3. Feedback to employees
   C. Conduct of performance appraisals
      1. Evaluation by immediate supervisor
      2. Frequency of evaluation

II. Evaluation principles
   A. Performance standards are behaviorally oriented
   B. Evaluation should be based on a representative behavioral sample
   C. Employee is given copies of evaluation related materials
      1. Job description
      2. Performance standards
      3. Evaluation form
   D. Documentation should include specific examples
   E. Prioritize areas of needed improvement
   F. Schedule evaluation time for convenience of both parties
   G. Structure conference to convey assistance

III. The evaluation tool
   A. Tool characteristics

1. Promote objectivity
   a. Objectivity defined
   b. Method of promoting objectivity
   c. Avoid "trigger" words
   d. Focus on actual job behaviors
2. Ensure validity
   a. Validity defined
   b. Methods of promoting validity
3. Ensure reliability
   a. Reliability defined
   b. Methods of promoting reliability

B. Types of evaluation devices
   1. Free response
   2. Ranking
   3. Checklist
   4. Graphic rating
   5. Forced choice comparison
   6. Behaviorally anchored rating scale

IV. Problems in performance appraisal
   A. Objectivity problems
      1. Halo effect
      2. Horns effect
   B. Interview conduct
      1. Principles in conducting appraisal interviews
      2. Manager behaviors
      3. Central tendency error
      4. Self aggrandizing effect

V. Management by objectives (MBO)
   A. Steps
   B. Performance objectives
      1. Development
      2. Examples
      3. Use
   C. Pros and cons of MBO evaluation
   D. Peer review

VI. Legal implications of performance appraisal
   A. Equal Pay Act
   B. Civil Rights Act
   C. Age Discrimination Employment Act
   D. Court decision examples

VII. Summary

GROUP PROJECT: Unit Manager Performance Evaluation Tool

In the following project students will practice chapter objectives 1, and 2.

Objective 1: Explain how a nurse manager should decide which behaviors to include on a staff nurse evaluation tool.

State responses to the above objective but specify behaviors expected of a unit manager.

Objective 2: Describe one advantage and one disadvantage of the following performance measuring devices:

a. Checklist
b. Ranking device
c. Rating scale
d. Free response form

Identify six applicable unit manager performance behaviors. Write sample tools for the performance behaviors using each of the following formats:

a. free response
b. ranking tool
c. checklist
d. graphic rating scale
e. forced choice comparison
f. behaviorally anchored rating scale

Text pages 539-541 may be used as a reference.

Objective 3: Indicate one method for increasing the reliability of a staff nurse performance-evaluation tool.

How might reliability be increased for the above tools?

CLASS ACTIVITY: Employee performance evaluation conference; role playing

The activity implements chapter objective 5: "Describe three actions that a head nurse could take to minimize a staff nurse's anxiety during her or his annual performance evaluation conference."

Select one student for the role of Nurse Unit Manager, and one student for the role of a staff nurse.

Situation

The Over 70s Nurse Unit Manager of Podville Hospital sends a memo to the probationary medical intensive care unit nurse telling her to report to the nurse unit manager's office at 2:00 pm Tuesday for an employee evaluation conference.

Questions

1. Critique the potential for positive effectiveness of the above action. (The students should identify the above as largely inappropriate.)

2. What should the nurse unit manager do to set up the employee evaluation conference to promote a more positive climate?

   (10 minutes)

Situation continued

The time for the employee conference has arrived. Have students assume the roles and role play the conference. Suggest to role players that they intentionally be inappropriate one or two times. Tell the class that the role players will intentionally be inappropriate at times. Allow the role players to play their part for about 10 minutes.

Questions

1. Have class critique the role playing:

   - identify interactions that could have been more constructive or positively presented.

   - state how the interactions identified could occur in a more constructive or positive way.

2. Have students identify positive interactions that occurred.

   (Faculty: students learn from both positive and negative examples, but be sure to turn each of the negatives into positives to leave all students with positive learning.)

TEST QUESTIONS

KNOWLEDGE AND COMPREHENSION

True : False

T F 29.01. The goal of the evaluation process is to improve employee performance.

T F 29.02. The most serious problem in performance appraisal is that some managers give *low* ratings to subordinates to demonstrate their own superior ability.

T F 29.03. The federal government defines employment practices as including selection, training, transfer, retention and promotion.

T F 29.04. Court decisions favor use of performance evaluation tools based upon systematic job analysis.

Matching: Match the type of evaluation device to the characteristic which best describes it. All answers will not be used.

Characteristics

___ 29.05. the nurse manager writes comments about the employee's performance

___ 29.06. the nurse manager designates the level of the employee's performance in relation to performance of other employees

___ 29.07. the nurse manager itemizes performance criteria and evaluates employee performance on each

___ 29.08. the nurse manager indicates the quality of the employee's performance by identifying a numerical value representing a performance level for each performance criteria

___ 29.09. The nurse manager chooses the descriptive statements which best and least describe the employer's performance.

Evaluation Devices

a. checklist

b. free respone form

c. forced choice comparison

d. ranking device on each

e. rating scale

f. BARS

Multiple Choice

29.10. Performance appraisal systems address which underlying factors?
1. employee ability
2. employee motivation
3. working environment
4. supervisory leadership style

a. 1, 2
b. 2, 3
c. 3, 4
d. all of above

29.11. When designing a performance evaluation tool the nurse manager will use which of the following to determine appropriate content?
a. job descriptions
b. performance standards
c. employee goals or objectives
d. all of above

29.12. Which of the following words will likely evoke emotional responses in the evaluator and should be avoided in the evaluation process?
1. disorganized
2. manipulative
3. argumentative
4. reliable

a. 1, 2
b. 2, 3
c. 3, 4
d. all of above

APPLICATION, ANALYSIS, AND/OR SYNTHESIS

29.13. To promote validity of the performance evaluation tool, Nurse manager C. Toit will:
1. verify currency of job description upon which the tool is based
2. verify that the tool contains categories in accordance to the position as it is actually practiced
3. ensure consistency of measurement when the tool is used by others
4. seek to design a simple, brief tool

a. 1, 2
b. 2, 3
c. 3, 4
d. all of above

29.14. To include management by objectives in the employee performance evaluation, Nurse manager C. Toit will do all of the following. In what order should she do them?
1. ask the employee to evaluate her own performance
2. negotiate goals
3. evaluate the employee
4. identify through consensus areas of need for improvement
5. meet to discuss the two evaluations

a. 1, 2, 3, 4, 5
b. 2, 3, 5, 4, 1
c. 1, 3, 5, 4, 2
d. 3, 2, 1, 5, 4

29.15. Which of the following is an appropriate interaction on the part of Nurse manager C. Toit during an employee evaluation conference?

a. "You seem to be quite argumentative with the nursing assistants."
b. "I'm concerned about your lack of reliability in regard to consistently finishing your assignments."
c. "It appears that you have met half of your goals for the writing of patient care standards."
d. all of above

29.16. The usually very competent staff nurse had made a major medication error two weeks prior to the evaluation. The unit manager rated the staff nurse below average through out the evaluation. The unit manager is exhibiting ?.

a. halo effect
b. horns effect
c. central tendency error
d. self-aggrandizement

26.17. The new unit manager who gave all of the unit's staff nurses very positive evaluations is exhibiting ?

a. halo effect
b. horns effect
c. central tendency error
d. self-aggrandizement

ANSWERS	TEXT REFERENCE
29.01. T	p. 538
29.02. b	p. 541
29.03. d	p. 545
29.04. a	p. 547
29.05. e	p. 539
29.06. d	p. 539
29.07. a	p. 539
29.08. c	p. 539, 540
29.09. c	p. 540
29.10. a	p. 536
29.11. d	p. 538
29.12. d	p. 538
29.13. a	p. 538, 539
29.14. c	p. 542, 543
29.15. c	p. 541, 542
29.16. b	p. 541
29.17. d	p. 541

CHAPTER

30

Discipline

The simple, basic instructions presented can guide the nurse manager in the appropriate use of disciplinary processes. Presentation of disciplinary actions as an educational experience for the employee aids the manager in attaining a useful perspective of the management process that includes control.

KEY TERMS

at will	transactional leaders
just cause	transformational leaders

OUTLINE

I. Discipline defined
   A. Employee's definition
   B. Manager's definition

II. Manager's right to discipline
   A. Institutional rules and regulations
   B. Collective bargaining agreements

III. Employee code of conduct
   A. Employee awareness
      1. Handbook
      2. "Postings"
   B. Examples
   C. Rationale for rules

IV. Disciplinary approach
   A. Traditional
   B. Developmental

V. Principles of discipline
   A. Purpose of discipline
   B. Rules/steps for correcting employees
      1. Promptly, privately, thoughtfully
      2. Progressive
         a. Counseling
         b. Verbal reprimand
         c. Written reprimand
         d. Suspension
         e. Discharge
      3. Thorough investigation
      4. Administer as aversive conditioning

VI. Dealing with disciplinary problems
   A. Sources of problems
      1. Method failure
      2. Procedural failure
   B. Disciplinary conference
      1. Conduct
      2. Content

3. Documentation
C. Disciplinary letter
    1. Reasons for
    2. Content of
    3. Record of
D. Errors in disciplining employees
    1. Delay in administering discipline
    2. Ignoring violation in hope that it is an isolated event
    3. Accumulation of rule violations, causing inappropriate manager responses
    4. Administering sweetened discipline
    5. Documentation failures
    6. Failure to follow rules and procedures
    7. Imposing discipline disproportionate to offense
    8. Disciplining inconsistently
E. Discipline as a teaching opportunity
F. Discharge
    1. At will
    2. Just cause
G. Positive discipline
    1. Description
    2. Steps

VII. Summary

GROUP PROJECT: Discipline for Nurse Idoit

The following activities incorporate chapter objectives 1, 2, and 3.

Objective 1: Describe the legal and organizational bases for a nurse manger's right to discipline a subordinate for unsatisfactory behavior.

Objective 2: Enumerate four employee behaviors that are considered "just cause" for disciple.

Objective 3: List six steps of progressive discipline in proper sequence and describe the nurse manager's responsibility at each step.

Time : 30 - 40 minutes

Setting: Home Health Care Agency "Kareall"

Situation

TUESDAY Home care nurse Idoit is a bright, aggressive, newly graduated ADN. Nursing manager Iam Wise is responsible for supervision of Ms. Idoit. Ms. Iam Wise received a phone call this morning from a patient relative stating that Ms. Idoit's manner with the patient left the patient in tears.

Question

In accordance with disciplinary principles presented in the text, how should Ms. Iam Wise respond to the patient relative?

(Expected responses at this point is the need to "hear" the problem; to concretely identify the offending behaviors; and to identify agency and/or contract policies and/or procedures which relate to the situation.)

THURSDAY Ms. Iam Wise decides to invoke the first step of the disciplinary process the next day.

Question

What will Ms. Iam Wise do?

(Expected responses include counseling with Nurse Idoit; giving Nurse Idoit opportunity to relate her perceptions of the situation; record the interaction.)

FRIDAY AM Nurse Idoit presents a very plausible picture of a family who refuses to challenge the patient to strive for improved health and less dependent function. Iam Wise decides to reassign Nurse Idoit to another family and to follow the progress of Nurse Idoit with the new family. Ms. Iam Wise will also monitor the progress of the patient under the auspices of another nurse. Ms. Iam Wise reminds Nurse Idoit of the agency philosophy that the ultimate authority for nursing care lies with the patient.

Question

Which disciplinary principles are being followed by Nurse Iam Wise on Thursday and Friday?

(Expected responses will include interaction with the employee in a timely manner; gathered information from both sides and will continue to gather relevant information; speaks to relevant agency philosophy/principles; uses situation to teach; initiates documentation.)

FRIDAY PM Nurse Iam Wise receives a patient satisfaction form from Nurse Idoit's first patient family. The patient's answer to the form question "Should you again need home care services, would you call us?" was a "NO!" On the bottom of the form the patient commented "Nurse pushy. Won't listen to me. Tried to design my life to suit her."

Friday was extremely busy and Nurse Iam Wise took no further action.

MONDAY Nurse Idoit burst into Nurse Iam Wise's office and demanded a change in assignment, "You just have to give me a different family. They don't need me."

Questions

1. What should Nurse Iam Wise do at this point?
2. Upon what principles/guidelines are these recommendations made?

CLASS ACTIVITY: Disciplinary conference role play

Time: 10-15 minutes for preparation for conference
10-15 minutes for role playing conference
follow-up discussion

Situation

The situation presented above with Nurse Idoit and Nurse Iam Wise is the basis for the role play. Utilize group responses to "Monday's" questions to have the class plan the conference.

Have students role play the conference per class plan.

Critique/discuss the role play:

- which principles presented in the text were applied?
- comment regarding verbal and nonverbal communications
- what influenced the effectiveness/outcome of the conference?
- how can Nurse Iam Wise help Nurse Idoit become a "positive" employee?
- what action(s) should Nurse Iam Wise now take?

CLASS DISCUSSION IDEA: Identifying "just cause" for employee discipline

The discussion implements chapter objectives 2 an 4:

Objective 2: Enumerate four employee behaviors that are considered "just cause" for discipline.

Objective 4: Identify at least four bases on which a manager's disciplinary action is apt to be reversed by an organizational superior or labor arbitrator.

1. Ask students to give examples of employee behaviors which would be "just cause" for discipline. (Experienced nurses will quickly see the value of having explicit institutional guidelines that apply to employee conduct.)
2. Using one of the "just cause" employee behaviors identified above, state actions Nurse manager Iam Wise will take to prevent reversal of potential future disciplinary action. (Expected responses will include thorough investigation and documentation of charges; follow "handbook" policy throughout; insuring employee awareness of rules and regulations; documenting progressive disciplinary steps.)

TEST QUESTIONS

KNOWLEDGE AND COMPREHENSION

True : False

T F 30.01 The basic prerequisite for effective discipline is employee awareness of agency rules and regulations governing employee behavior.

T F 30.02 The nurse manager should wait until the staff nurse has opportunity to calm down before disciplining her.

T F 30.03 To be effective, discipline should be administered as punishment.

Multiple Choice

30.04. Which of the following provide a basis for the nurse manager to discipline a subordinate?
a. collective bargaining agreements
b. agency rules and regulations
c. agency codes of conduct
d. all of above

30.05. The primary goal of developmental disciplinary procedures is to:
a. punish employees exhibiting inappropriate behavior
b. educate problem employees
c. improve employee performance
d. all of above

30.06. Each of the following are progressive disciplinary actions. Choose the order in which they should be practiced.
1. counseling
2. discharge
3. longer suspension
4. short suspension
5. verbal reprimand
6. written reprimand
a. 1, 4, 3, 6, 5, 2
b. 1, 5, 6, 4, 3, 2
c. 5, 1, 6, 4, 3, 2
d. 5, 6, 1, 4, 5, 2

30.07. Which of the following should be a focus of an employee disciplinary conference?
a. explanation of the broken rule
b. examples of inappropriate employee actions
c. expected employee behavioral change
d. all of above

30.08. Discipline is warranted if the:
a. employee was inappropriate in behavior
b. employee realized she was breaking a rule
c. employee wanted to follow older procedure
d. all of above

30.09. An employee who is terminated in a manner that violates rights may claim:
a. "at will" rule
b. "for cause" rule
c. wrongful discharge
d. all of above

30.10. An employer who terminates an employee for no cause is practicing:
a. "at will" rule
b. "for cause" rule
c. wrongful discharge
d. positive discipline

APPLICATION, ANALYSIS, AND/OR SYNTHESIS

Multiple Choice

30.11. When Nurse Iam Wise counsels Nurse Idoit regarding inappropriate nurse behaviors toward the patient and the patient family, Nurse Iam Wise must first ensure that:
  a. agency standards of conduct for nurses includes nurse:patient relationships
  b. all relevant facts have been gathered prior to conference
  c. the union representative is invited to attend the session
  d. all of above

30.12. Which of the following would usually be considered "just cause" for disciplining an employee?
  a. Nurse Ine Briate arrived on the unit late, walked with an unsteady gait, spoke with slurred speech, and her breath smelled of alcohol
  b. Nurse Iam Purfect charted a treatment as being done which neither she nor the staff she was supervising had performed
  c. Nurse Myown Mind refuses to perform certain tasks that are a part of her job description
  d. all of above

30.13. Which of the following would be reason to counsel an employee as the first step of disciplinary action?
  a. When the unit was particularly hectic, Nurse Iva Hadit shouted abusively at an aggressive, hindering family member.
  b. Nurse Hon Gree left the unit to get a snack without telling anyone.
  c. Nurse Cantbe Bothered consistently wears dirty shoes, and neglects to wear her hospital name tag
  d. all of above

30.14. Agency personnel policies and procedures require progressive disciplinary practices; a written warning, followed by a three-day suspension and final written warning, and discharge. Nurse manager I. Goofed discharged the nurse subordinate Notsogood without first suspending Nurse Notsogood. What would be the expected outcome of this action?
  a. Nurse Notsogood is no longer with the agency.
  b. Nurse manager I. Goofed is relieved of her position.
  c. Nurse Notsogood is rehired following a grievance process.
  d. Nurse staff morale improves following the dismissal of Nurse Notsogood.

30.15. Which of the following would be the most appropriate statement for a nurse manager to make during an employee disciplinary conference?
  a. "Your attitude toward the patients is inappropriate."
  b. "Three times this week the discharge process has not been followed for patients you have discharged."
  c. "If you cannot improve your working relationship with the nursing assistants, I will have to put you on suspension."
  d. "You seem to want more authority and have been trying to control the assignments of other staff nurses."

30.16. Which of the following would likely lead to a reversal of a decision to discharge an employee whose behavior was inappropriate?

a. Several RNs delegated a RN task to nursing assistants. One of the RNs was discharged for this practice.
b. A treatment procedure was mishandled by the nurse resulting in a patient infection. The nurse was reinstructed regarding inappropriate treatment procedure. The nurse was discharged when she subsequently continued to practice the procedure inappropriately.
c. A report of an incident, counsel about the incident, and repeated occurrence of the incident were filed in the personnel file with copies given to the employee.
d. All of the above

ANSWERS	TEXT REFERENCE
30.01. T	p. 551
30.02. F	p. 553
30.03. F	p. 553
30.04. d	p. 550
30.05. c	p. 551
30.06. b	p. 551-553
30.07. d	p. 553-554
30.08. b	p. 553
30.09. c	p. 556
30.10. a	p. 556
30.11. a	p. 551
30.12. d	p. 551-553
30.13. c	p. 552, 553
30.14. c	p. 555
30.15. b	p. 553-554
30.16. a	p. 555

CHAPTER

31

Law

In the text summary for this chapter, the author has succinctly stated the responsibility of the nurse manager in regard to the law: ". . . to become sufficiently informed about nursing practice conditions in the agency or unit and about laws governing nursing and management to protect herself or himself, subordinates, and employer from personal, professional, and economic losses from malpractice." (page 576) With this responsibility in mind, the student can pursue this readable chapter to gain a legal awareness that can aid him/her in management practices that will lead to preventive management practices. Preventing legal contention is an astute and significant management goal.

KEY TERMS

administrative law
assault
battery
civil law
common law
defamation
false imprisonment
law
living will
malpractice
negligence
patient's consent
revocation
right to privacy
sexual harassment
slander
statutory law
suspension

OUTLINE

I. Overview
   A. Law defined
   B. American law
      1. Civil
      2. Criminal

II. Origins of law
   A. Sources
      1. Statutory
      2. Common
      3. Administrative
   B. Changing law
   C. Application

III. The nurse as employee
   A. Licensure
      1. Defined
      2. Mandatory licensure
      3. Permissive licensure
      4. Purpose
      5. Nursing licensure board
   B. Definition of nursing in nursing licensure acts
      1. General definition in nursing acts
      2. ANA guidelines
      3. Determining legality of nurse practice
   C. Requirements for licensure
      1. Common state requirements

a. Minimum age
b. Citizenship
c. Good moral character
d. Approved formal education
e. Examination
2. Licensing out-of-state nurses
a. Reciprocity
b. Endorsement
c. Waiver
d. Examination
3. "Graduate" nurse practice
D. Suspension and revocation of license
1. Suspension defined
2. Revocation
a. Defined
b. Causes
E. Employee's rights
F. Civil rights
1. Basis of rights
2. Protection against wrongful discharge
3. Allowed exceptions
G. Occupational safety and health act
H. Responsibility for appointing and assigning personnel
1. Implementation of institutional policies
2. Temporary staffing obligations
I. Responsibility for quality control
1. Responsibility of nursing administration
2. Duties
a. Observe
b. Report
c. Correct
3. Verification of identification and credentials
4. Protection against drug impaired employees
a. Incidence
b. Drug testing
J. Sexual harassment
1. Definition
2. EEOC guidelines
3. Employer responsibility
K. Worker's Compensation laws

IV. The nurse's responsibility to patients
A. Negligence
1. Definition
2. Malpractice
a. Definition
b. Standard of care
c. Examples
3. Evidence of nursing negligence
4. Impact of expertise
5. Negligence examples
6. Malpractice examples
B. False imprisonment
1. Definition
2. Restraint parameters
a. Self protection
b. Protection from others
c. Suicide prevention policy
C. Good Samaritan laws
D. Responsibility for equipment
1. Equipment is functional
2. Equipment is correctly operated
E. Right to privacy
1. Content
2. Privacy
a. Definition
b. Examples
c. Manager's responsibility
F. Informed consent
1. Description
2. Assault and battery
3. Content
4. Procedure
5. Written or tape recorded
6. Therapeutic nondisclosure
G. Confidential communications
1. Description
2. Uses
H. Responsibility for observation and reporting
1. Legal obligation
2. Prompt recording and reporting

V. Advance care directives
A. Patient self determination
B. Types
1. Living will
2. Durable power of attorney
3. Advance care medical directive
C. Values history

VI. The nurse's relationship to the physician
A. Legal perspective
1. "Respondent superior"
2. "Borrowed servant"
3. Independent nurse
B. Sponge, instrument, and needle counts
1. JCAHO guideline
2. Nurse responsibility
C. Standing orders
1. Limitation
2. Definition
3. Responsibility
D. Clarification of treatment and discharge orders

1. Suitability of order
2. Nonconcurrence with manufacturers' recommendations
3. Inappropriateness of discharge

E. Oral orders
1. Procedural policy
2. Conditions

F. Responsibility to protect patient from harm

G. Slander, libel, and character assassination
1. Defamation
2. Slander
3. Complaint process

VII. The nurse's responsibility to protect the public

VIII. Nurse's responsibility for record keeping and reporting

A. Patient's medical record
1. Description
2. Property rights
3. Failure to record
4. Correcting errors
5. Falsifying records

B. Reporting public health information

IX. Summary

GROUP ACTIVITY: Preventing legal problems through policies and procedures

The activity potentially contributes to each chapter objective.

Time: 30 minutes plus discussion time

Divide class into three or more small groups

- one group is to assume the position of Nurse unit manager of Podville Hospital's Over 70s unit
- one group is to assume the position of a Nurse unit manager of Podville's Longterm Care Facility. The unit is oriented toward "shorter" term stay patients with greater medical and skilled nursing needs.
- one group is to assume the position of a Nurse Manager of Podville's Home Care Agency. The focus of the agency is to provide supportive and rehabilitative services which assist patients in continuing to live in their own homes in contrast to being institutionalized.

Activity

The effective nurse manager wants to practice preventive management. You as a nurse manager are to identify areas of potential legal concern which can be addressed through policies and/or procedures. Using Chapter 31 of the text as a resource, list three policies and/or procedures for each of the following:

(1) nurses as employees
(2) nurse relationships
(3) nurse practice

as they relate to the nature of the services for which you are responsible.

DISCUSSION IDEA: Hiring practices and the law

Discussion can incorporate chapter objectives 2 and 3.

Objective 2: Enumerate three requirements for nursing licensure that are specified by statute in most states.

Objective 3: Explain how Title VII of the Civil Rights Act of 1964 relates to the hiring of staff nurses.

Preparation

1. Obtain a copy of hiring procedures used by a facility with which students are familiar. Reproduce them for students or copy onto overheads.

2. Obtain a copy of state nursing licensure statutes.

Questions

1. How are the provisions of Title VII of the Civil Rights Act of 1964 incorporated in the hiring procedures/practices?

2. What specific requirements regarding nursing licensure are included? What do the state statutes require?

3. Are there recommendations the class would make in light of the above?

DISCUSSION: Laws governing nursing practice.

Time: 10 minutes

Use objective 1 as a discussion topic.

Objective 1: Cite one example of statutory law, one example of case law, and one example of administrative law that governs nursing practice.

DISCUSSION: Workmen's Compensation

Time: 10 minutes

Objective 4 may also be used as a discussion topic.

Objective 4: Explain two conditions that must be met for a nurse claimant to obtain compensation under a state's Workmen's Compensation law.

TEST QUESTIONS

KNOWLEDGE AND COMPREHENSION

True : False

T F 31.01. Nurse managers at all levels are legally obligated to ensure nursing care quality.

T F 31.02. Federal law requires medical personnel to tell the inquiring patient complete information about diagnosis and treatment.

T F 31.03. The patient has a eight to information contained in the medical record.

Matching: Match the type of law to the description by placing the appropriate letter in the space provided.

	Description	Type of Law
____ 31.04.	legal principles evolving from court decisions	a. administrative law
____ 31.05.	enactments of federal and state legislative bodies	b. common law
____ 31.06.	rules and regulations of agencies appointed by the executive branch of government	c. statutory law
____ 31.07.	State Health Department codes	

Matching: Match the Act/Law to its focus by placing the appropriate letter in the space provided.

Focus

____ 31.08. forbids discrimination on the basis of race, religion, sex or national origin

____ 31.09. protects employment rights of persons between the ages of 40 and 65 years

____ 31.10. assure safe and healthful working conditions for working men and women

____ 31.11. provides a legal means for obtaining compensation for illness or injuries suffered during employment

____ 31.12. provides that written information about the right to make decisions about medical care be given Medicare and Medicaid patients at time of admission

____ 31.13. exempt nurses from liabilities when they render first aid to persons in emergencies

Act/Law

a. Age Discrimination in Employment Act of 1967

b. Good Samaritan laws

c. Occupational Safety and Health Act of 1970

d. Patient Self Determination Act

e. Title VII of the Civil Rights

f. Workmen's Compensation

Multiple Choice

31.14. Which of the following best represents the primary purpose of nursing licensure laws?
a. to improve the quality of nursing practice
b. to protect the public through enforcement of minimum standards
c. to provide a standard of excellence for nursing practice
d. all of above

31.15. Most state nursing licensure laws include:
a. provision for license suspension
b. definition of nursing
c. licensure requirements
d. all of above

31.16. Most state nursing licensure statutes specify which of the following personal characteristics as requirements for nursing licensure?
a. drug free, entry level competencies, passage of examination
b. minimum of 21 years of age, U.S. citizenship, good moral character
c. educational reference, interview, passage of examination
d. all of above

31.17. An advance care medical directive:
   a. establishes care nurses can give in an emergency when physician is not available
   b. combines a living will and durable power of attorney for health care
   c. identifies legal standards of medical practice
   d. none of above

31.18. The operating room nurse on duty when a sponge was accidentally left in the patient's body will probably be found:
   a. liable
   b. guilty of defamation
   c. guilty of battery
   d. none of above

APPLICATION, ANALYSIS, AND/OR SYNTHESIS

Matching: Match the legal problem to the incident that demonstrates the problem by placing the appropriate letter in the space provided.

	Incident	Legal Problem
___	31.19. The unit was short staffed so the nurses used restraint belts on all patients over 65 years who were up.	a. battery
		b. defamation
___	31.20. Although the facility policy requires that two persons transport a patient, only one nurse took the patient to x-ray and the patient was injured when he rolled off the cart	c. false imprisonment
		d. invasion of privacy
		e. negligence
___	31.21. The male patient charged that he was a victim of the female nurse who catheterized him without his permission.	
___	31.22. The nurse told a visitor that his friend has AIDS	
___	31.23. The emergency room nurse told the patient that the physician the patient requested was not a good one to treat the injury. The physician threatens to sue the nurse on what basis?	

Multiple Choice

31.24. Nurse Klutz contacted hepatitis B by puncturing herself with a needle that had been used to give a hepatitis B patient IV medication. The employer will be required to pay compensation to Nurse Klutz because of provisions in the:

a. Good Samaritan Law
b. Occupational Safety and Health Act of 1970
c. Workmen's Compensation laws
d. Civil Rights Act of 1964

31.25. The state health department guidelines specify that an AIDS patient may be housed in a double room if his/her condition does not otherwise merit a private room. A family sues the hospital nursing staff for moving their loved one into a room with an AIDS patient. The hospital nursing staff is likely to be:

a. found not negligent
b. found negligent
c. guilty of malpractice
d. not guilty of malpractice

ANSWERS	TEXT REFERENCE
31.01. T	p. 565
31.02. F	p. 570
31.03. T	p. 574
31.04. b	p. 561
31.05. c	p. 560,561
31.06. a	p. 561
31.07. a	p. 561
31.08. e	p. 564
31.09. a	p. 564
31.10. c	p. 564
31.11. f	p. 566
31.12. d	p. 570, 571
31.13. b	p. 568
31.14. b	p. 561
31.15. d	p. 561, 562
31.16. b	p. 562
31.17. b	p. 571
31.18. a	p. 569, 572, 574
31.19. c	p. 568
31.20. e	p. 567
31.21. a	p. 569
31.22. d	p. 569
31.23. b	p. 574
31.24. c	p. 566
31.25. a	p. 567

CHAPTER

32

Labor-Management Relations

The nursing manager can gain an overview of management-labor history, relationships, and conduct from this chapter. The exercises in this *Manual* will challenge the nurse who has nonmanagerial experience with unions to view contract outcomes from a different perspective, identifying both the positive and the limiting outcomes of collective bargaining.

KEY TERMS

grievance   strike   union decertification

OUTLINE

I. Definitions
  A. Labor
  B. Labor force
  C. Managers
  D. Relationships
  E. Union or labor organization

II. Collective bargaining
  A. Chief activities
    1. Collective bargaining
      a. Rule making
      b. Negotiations
    2. Conflict resolution
  B. Labor agreement
    1. Definition
    2. Use
  C. Wagner Act/National Labor Relations Act
    1. Right to union
    2. National Labor Relations Board
  D. Taft-Hartley Act/Labor-Management Relations Act
    1. Reaffirmed collective bargaining rights
    2. Limited collective bargaining activities
  E. ANA's Economic Security Program
  F. Amendments to 1974 Taft-Hartley Act
    1. 10 days' strike notice
    2. 90 days' termination notice
  G. Proliferation of collective bargaining groups
  H. Opposition to collective bargaining

III. History of labor organization
  A. Overview
  B. Violence
  C. Post World War II
    1. Entry into health industry

IV. Reasons for unionization by nurses
  A. Higher salaries, increased benefits
  B. Improve working conditions
  C. Control practice conditions
  D. Strike

1. Defined
2. Occurrence

E. Future issues

V. Characteristics of labor unions
   A. Political institution
   B. Union certification
   C. Defining membership
      1. Certification process
      2. Definition of supervisor
         a. Taft-Hartley Act definition
         b. ANA definition

VI. Management and unionization
   A. Administrative viewpoint
   B. Cautions
   C. Managerial rights

VII. Preparation for collective bargaining
   A. Management preparation
      1. Establish/maintain pleasant relationship
      2. Be aware of labor negotiations in other facilities
      3. Analyze recurring grievances and supervisory problems
      4. Know wage-salary structures of other facilities
      5. Be aware of National Labor Relations Act content
         a. Prohibited management actions
         b. Prohibited union actions
      6. Solicitation of membership
      7. Identify positions represented by union
   B. Negotiating team
      1. Appointed by hospital administrator and union president
         a. Labor lawyer as hospital's spokesperson
         b. Labor lawyer or experienced negotiator as union spokes person
      2. Role of director of nursing
      3. Preparation of hospital's spokesperson

VIII. Contract negotiations
   A. Roles of negotiating team members
   B. Adversarial relationship
   C. Conduct of bargaining talks
   D. Bargaining in good faith
   E. Sequence of events

IX. Negotiating principles
   1. Deliberate one issue at a time
   2. Explore all issues before reaching final agreement on any one issue
   3. Ask full explanation for requested changes
   4. Firmly resist demands that are objectionable to management
   5. Adhere firmly to agreed upon principles
   6. Emphasize facts
   7. Use processes for keeping "cool"
   8. Keep log of negotiations
   9. Identify mandatory, permissible, and nonbargainable issues
   10. Present data pertaining to unreasonable demands
   11. Reject unacceptable position
   12. Avoid trials of strength
   13. Upon agreement, initial, and set issue aside
   14. Methods to avoid breakdown
   15. Keep nonunion supervisory personnel informed of progress
   16. Analyze proposals in terms of patients' needs, staffing resources, institutional policies, and management strategy
   17. When talks break down utilize a fact finder

X. Contract ratification
   A. Verify final draft
   B. Ratify contract with total membership

XI. Contract administration
   A. Roles of nurse managers
   B. Grievance procedures
      1. Grievance defined
      2. Four steps of grievance procedure
      3. Focus of grievances
      4. Principles to determine fairness of grieved issue

XII. Decertification
   A. Reason for
   B. Process

XIII. Summary

ASSIGNMENT: Impact of nursing contract provisions

The assignment incorporates chapter objective 5.

Objective 5: List three issues designated by the National Labor Relations Board as mandatory issues for collective bargaining between union and management.

Activity

Interview a registered nurse in a staff nurse position in a facility which has a negotiated contract. Include the questions listed below in the interview.

Interview a nurse manager in the same facility. Use the same questions. (Do make sure that the nurse manager has responsibility for all aspects of staffing.)

Questions

1. What issues in the contract have contributed to your satisfaction with your current job?
2. Do any issues in the contract contribute to your dissatisfaction with your job?
3. When the contract comes up for renewal, would you prefer to be nonunionized?

   If yes, why?

   If no, what issues should be negotiated which would contribute to increased job satisfaction?

In three to five typed page:

1. Briefly describe each of the interviewees in relation to their respective positions.
2. State interviewee responses to each question.
3. Compare the responses of the staff nurse and the nurse manager. Do they view the contract differently?
4. Which of the issues identified in the interviews are:
   - mandatory issues
   - permissible issues
   - nonbargainable issue?

CLASS DISCUSSION IDEA: Contracts - two sides of the coin

Nursing management often views collective bargaining as a "mixed blessing." Both positive and negative aspects are concurrent. For the following negotiated items draw from the class *both* potential positive and negative outcomes for each item as perceived by a nurse manager.

1. Wages are increased to amounts that are greater than those paid by comparative facilities in the area.
2. Nurses are to be granted every other weekend off.
3. Nurses may work no more than 80 hours in a two week pay period without receiving time-and-a-half pay.
4. Benefits remain as previously negotiated.

CLASSROOM GROUP ACTIVITY: Negotiating

The activity will include chapter objectives 1, 2, 4, and 5.

Objective 1: Describe two unfair labor practices by management (as defined by the National Labor Relations Act).

Objective 2: Describe two unfair labor practices by a union (as defined by the National Labor Relations Act).

Objective 4: Recommend three actions to be taken by an agency's vice-president of nursing and nurse administrators when preparing to negotiate a contract with the inion that represents agency nurses.

Objective 5: List three issues designated by the National labor Relations Board as mandatory issues for collective bargaining between union and management.

Time: 1 class period

Situation: Nursing contracts for RNs, LPNs, and nursing assistants will expire in two months.

Preliminary proposals were rejected by the union membership.

Staff concerns:
RNs are concerned with practice issues.
LPNs are feeling threatened as LPN positions are being filled with RNs and want job security.
Nursing assistants want higher hourly wages and more week ends off.

Management concerns:
Management is experiencing considerable budget constraint and cash flow problems. Management has found that LPNs are no longer cost:benefit effective.

Assign students to one of three groups:
- 5-10 students to represent management
- 5-10 students to represent nursing staff
- remaining students to critique group.

Preparation: Instruct both management and nursing staff groups to:
- purposefully role play one unfair labor practice.
- identify negotiators
- identify negotiating team
- in addition management is to identify two unacceptable positions.

Role play

Faculty role is to stimulate all class members to participate. Faculty will want to tell the critique group that they are to identify any unfair labor practices which occur.

Seat negotiating teams in front of the class and ask the critique group what the first step for the negotiating meeting should be. Play out for 10-15 minutes or until unfair labor practices have occurred on both sides.

Discuss what happened, why it is disallowed, and what approach could have prevented the unfair labor practices.

Ask the critique group to identify the behaviors which facilitated positive negotiations.

Classify the identified issues.

TEST QUESTIONS

KNOWLEDGE AND COMPREHENSION

True : False

T F 32.01. The National Labor Relations Act of 1935 effectively protected labor leaving management at a disadvantage.

T F 32.02. The Taft-Hartley Act specified that supervisors could be part of the bargaining unit.

T F 32.03. Labor law now specifies that a 10 day notice must be given before striking a health agency.

T F 32.04. In the future, the primary reason for nurses to join a labor organization will likely be to negotiate regarding professional concerns.

T F 32.05. During union negotiation meetings the nurse administrator should strongly present nursing needs.

Multiple Choice

32.06. Which of the following working conditions would contribute to a decision for nurses to unionize?
a. competitive salaries
b. decentralized decision making
c. limited advancement opportunity
d. all of above

32.07. Which of the following are mandated collective bargaining issues?
a. wages
b. hours
c. terms and conditions of employment
d. all of above

32.08. Which of the following characterize labor unions?
a. relationships between management and unions are adversarial
b. operates as a political institution
c. once certified, the union has exclusive bargaining rights.
d. all of above

32.09. When labor contract negotiations break down both parties may agree to arbitration. Which of the following best represents a commitment to arbitration?
a. The arbitrator will present recommendations, which the parties are free to accept or reject.
b. The arbitrator will present facts and rationale and act as moderator during discussion and resolution by the parties.
c. The arbitrator will present his decision which both parties will follow.
d. Any one of the above, as determined at the time.

32.10. When labor contract negotiations break down both parties may agree to use a fact finder. The commitment to using a fact finder means that:
a. The fact finder will present recommendations, which the parties are free to accept or reject.
b. The fact finder will present facts and rationale and act as moderator during discussion and resolution by the parties.
c. The arbitrator will present his decision which both parties will follow.
d. Any one of the above, as determined at the time.

APPLICATION, ANALYSIS, AND/OR SYNTHESIS

Multiple Choice

32.11. Which of the following nursing management actions would be considered as fair labor practice by management?
a. The director of nursing encourages all newly employed nurses to join the state nurses' association which bargains for the nurses.
b. The director of nursing honors a request for a paid staff development day for a union member to receive collective bargaining training?
c. The director of nursing identifies positions which qualify as supervisory positions.
d. The director of nursing asks the secretary to schedule a room and time for union members to meet.

32.12. Which of the following actions of a nurse manager would be considered grounds for a grievance?
a. A nurse was promoted on the basis of ability rather than on the basis of seniority as specified in the contract.
b. When the new supervisor was hired she was told that hospital policy requires that she not be an ANA member.
c. The nursing administrator insisted that he implement established disciplinary procedures for a problem nurse employee.
d. The nursing administrator overrode a unit recommendation to promote a staff nurse.

32.13. Which of the following would be (an) unfair labor practice(s) by a union representing nurses at Podville Hospital.
a. The union declared that the membership would go on strike in five days.
b. The union notified administration that they want to modify the bargaining agreement next month.
c. The union insists that Podville Hospital's nurse unit managers, who have full responsibility for all aspects of staffing their units, be included in union membership.
d. all of above

32.14. When the union representative obtained support of 25 percent of the employed nurses, he presented a memo to administration that his union would subsequently be representing the nurses of the facility. The administrator should:
a. recognize the union as the official bargaining agent for the nurses
b. reply to the union representative that the union cannot represent the nurses at this time
c. meet with the nurses to verify their intent to unionize
d. meet with the nurses to resolve dissatisfactions

32.15. Which of the following best represents the role of the director of nursing in preparation for collective bargaining?
a. The director of nursing has no role in contract negotiations between a union representing nurses and hospital administration.
b. When negotiations have begun she should follow the issues.
c. Determine positions represented by the union and the number of personnel occupying the positions.
d. Prepare arguments that represent management needs for her presentation during negotiations.

32.16. In which of the following situations would it be appropriate for the nurse to ask the union to represent her in presenting a grievance?
a. The staff nurse was not granted a special leave request.
b. The staff nurse was not granted a raise on the basis of a poor performance evaluation.
c. The staff nurse is scheduled for orientation and assignment to another unit after her primary unit is closed.
d. all of above

ANSWERS	TEXT REFERENCE
32.01. T	p. 580
32.02. F	p. 580
32.03. T	p. 581
32.04. T	p. 582
32.05. F	p. 587
32.06. c	p. 582
32.07. d	p. 580
32.08. d	p. 583
32.09. c	p. 589, 590
32.10. a	p. 589
32.11. c	p. 583, 584
32.12. a	p. 590
32.13. d	p. 585, 586
32.14. b	p. 583
32.15. c	p. 585
32.16. b	p. 580, 590, 591

Figures

FIGURE 1.1

RELATIONSHIP OF MANAGEMENT PROCESS TO NURSING PROCESS

NURSING PROCESS	MANAGEMENT PROCESS
ASSESSING	SITUATIONAL ASSESSMENT
DIAGNOSING	IDENTIFYING PROBLEMS
PLANNING	PLANNING • Establishing objectives, policies, procedures • Organizing
IMPLEMENTING	DIRECTING OTHERS: • Leading, communicating, motivating
EVALUATING	EVALUATING • Preventing • Controlling

NOTE: EACH OF THESE PROCESSES IS CYCLICAL

FIGURE 3.1

RELATIONSHIPS OF AGENCY AND NURSING DEPARTMENT STRUCTURES

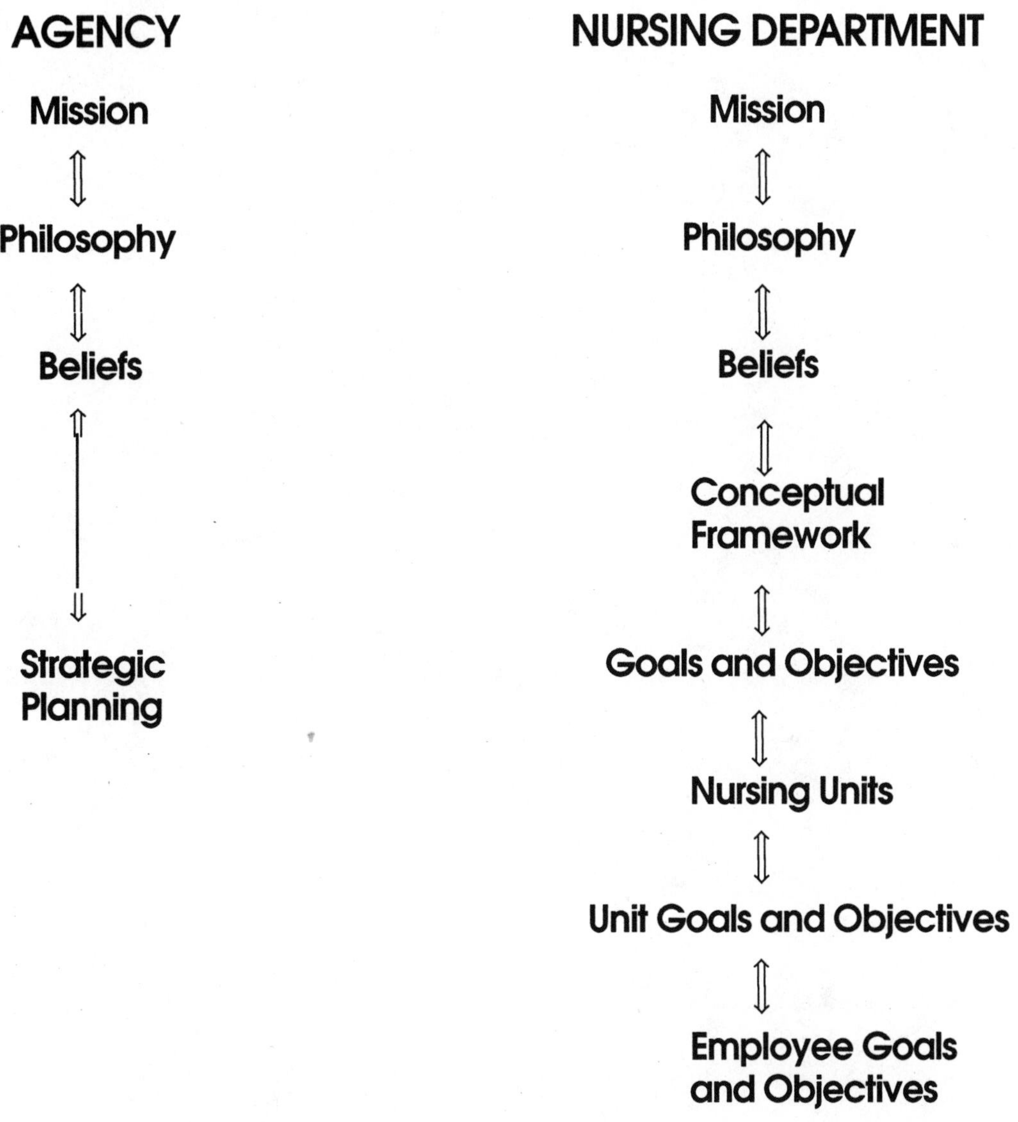

Note: Ideally all relationships are bidirectional.

FIGURE 6.1

RELATIONSHIPS OF NURSING STANDARDS TO SYSTEMS THEORY AND MANAGEMENT PROCESS

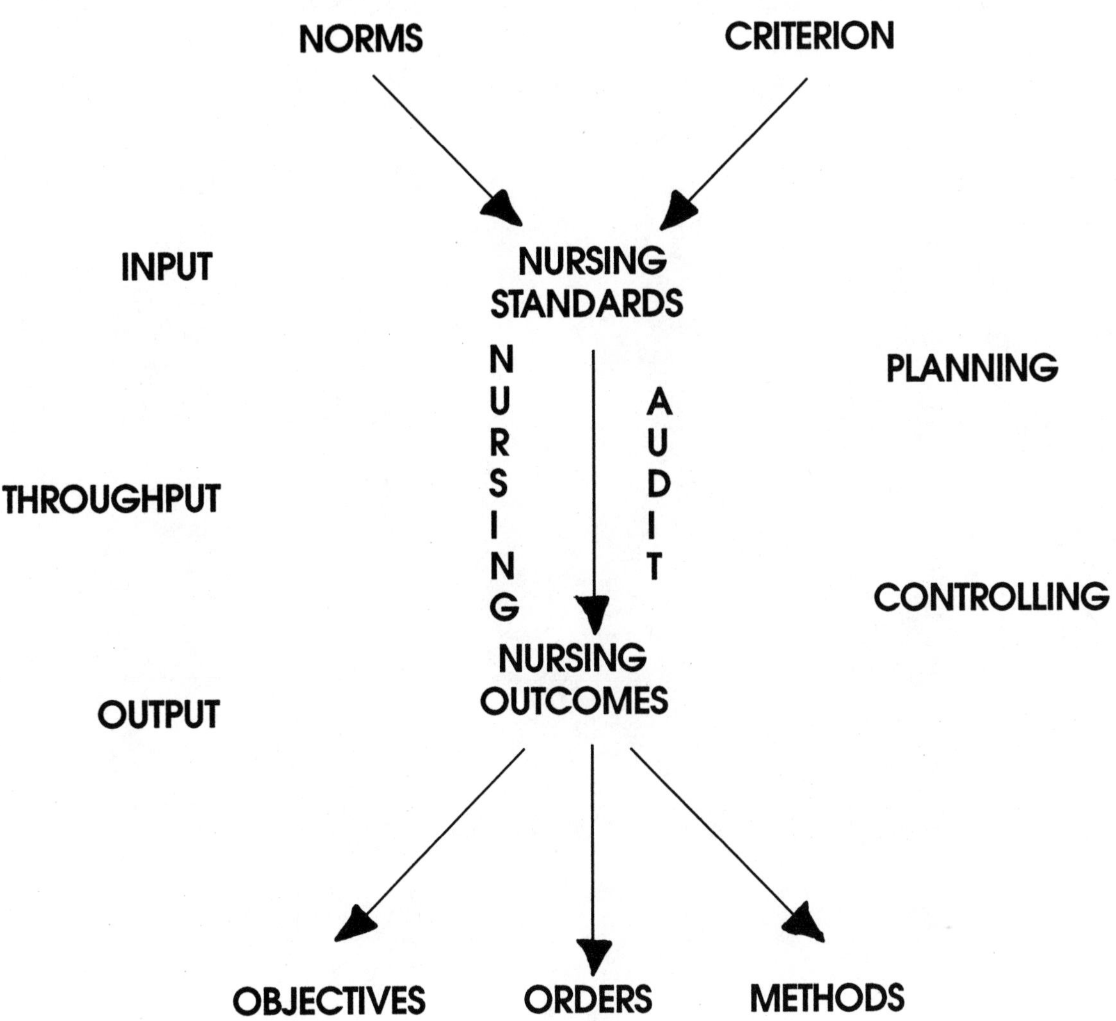

FIGURE 7.1
PODVILLE HOSPITAL ORGANIZATIONAL CHART

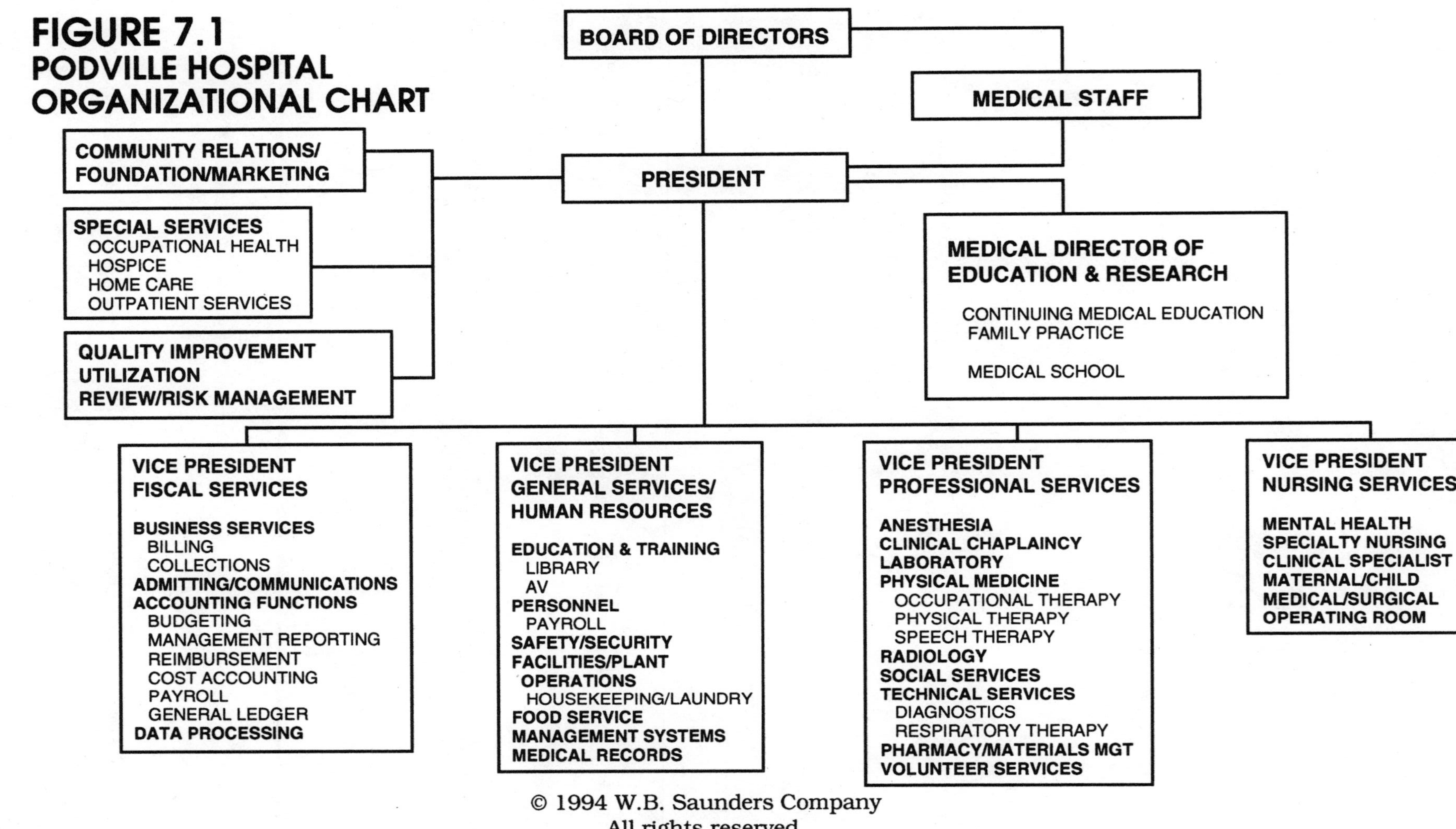

BOARD OF DIRECTORS
MEDICAL STAFF
PRESIDENT
COMMUNITY RELATIONS/ FOUNDATION/MARKETING
SPECIAL SERVICES
OCCUPATIONAL HEALTH
HOSPICE
HOME CARE
OUTPATIENT SERVICES
QUALITY IMPROVEMENT
UTILIZATION
REVIEW/RISK MANAGEMENT
MEDICAL DIRECTOR OF EDUCATION & RESEARCH
CONTINUING MEDICAL EDUCATION
FAMILY PRACTICE
MEDICAL SCHOOL
VICE PRESIDENT FISCAL SERVICES
BUSINESS SERVICES
BILLING
COLLECTIONS
ADMITTING/COMMUNICATIONS
ACCOUNTING FUNCTIONS
BUDGETING
MANAGEMENT REPORTING
REIMBURSEMENT
COST ACCOUNTING
PAYROLL
GENERAL LEDGER
DATA PROCESSING
VICE PRESIDENT GENERAL SERVICES/ HUMAN RESOURCES
EDUCATION & TRAINING
LIBRARY
AV
PERSONNEL
PAYROLL
SAFETY/SECURITY
FACILITIES/PLANT OPERATIONS
HOUSEKEEPING/LAUNDRY
FOOD SERVICE
MANAGEMENT SYSTEMS
MEDICAL RECORDS
VICE PRESIDENT PROFESSIONAL SERVICES
ANESTHESIA
CLINICAL CHAPLAINCY
LABORATORY
PHYSICAL MEDICINE
OCCUPATIONAL THERAPY
PHYSICAL THERAPY
SPEECH THERAPY
RADIOLOGY
SOCIAL SERVICES
TECHNICAL SERVICES
DIAGNOSTICS
RESPIRATORY THERAPY
PHARMACY/MATERIALS MGT
VOLUNTEER SERVICES
VICE PRESIDENT NURSING SERVICES
MENTAL HEALTH
SPECIALTY NURSING
CLINICAL SPECIALIST
MATERNAL/CHILD
MEDICAL/SURGICAL
OPERATING ROOM

FIGURE 7.2
PODVILLE HOSPITAL
NURSING DEPARTMENT

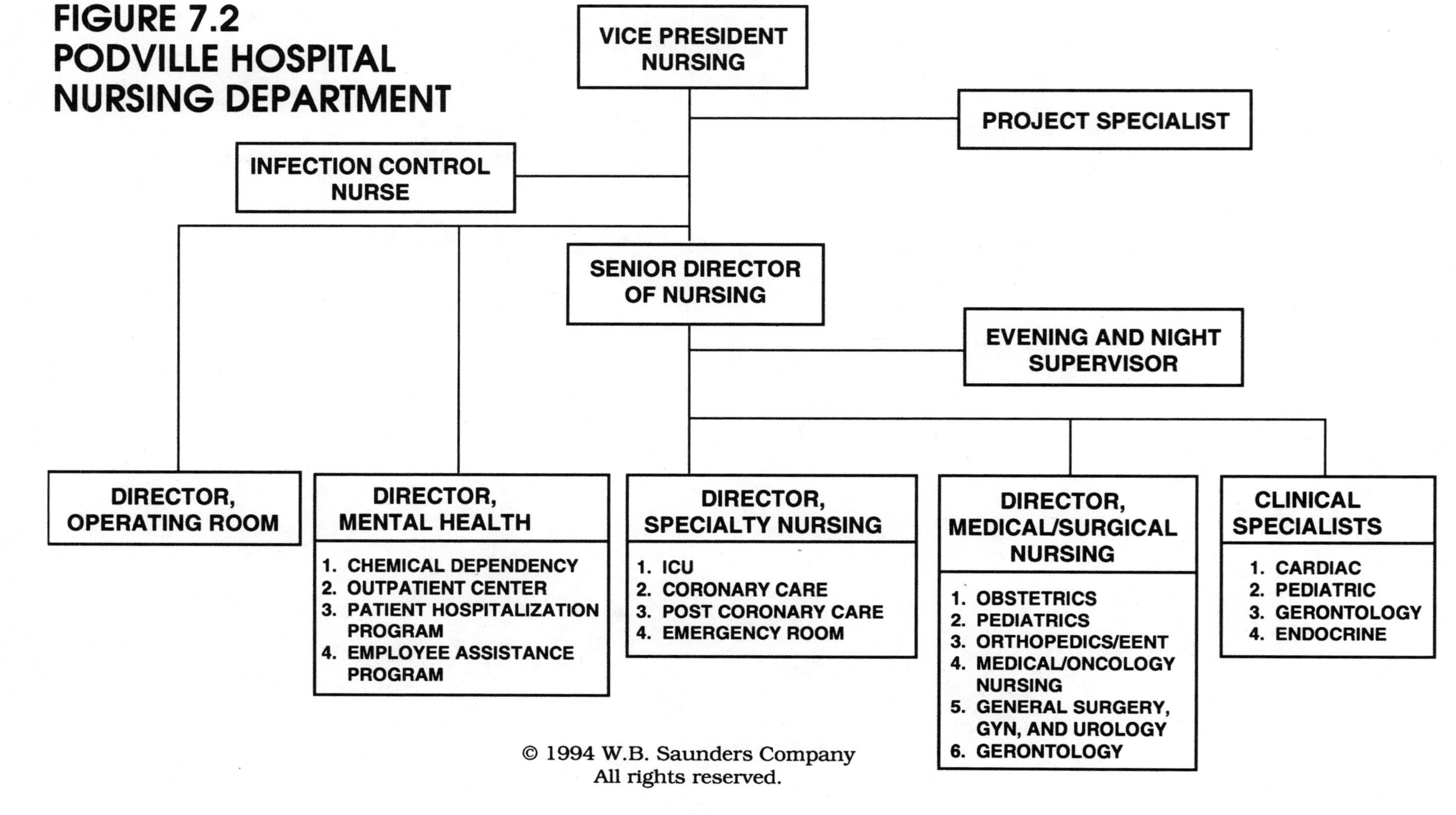
VICE PRESIDENT NURSING
PROJECT SPECIALIST
INFECTION CONTROL NURSE
SENIOR DIRECTOR OF NURSING
EVENING AND NIGHT SUPERVISOR
DIRECTOR, OPERATING ROOM
DIRECTOR, MENTAL HEALTH
1. CHEMICAL DEPENDENCY
2. OUTPATIENT CENTER
3. PATIENT HOSPITALIZATION PROGRAM
4. EMPLOYEE ASSISTANCE PROGRAM
DIRECTOR, SPECIALTY NURSING
1. ICU
2. CORONARY CARE
3. POST CORONARY CARE
4. EMERGENCY ROOM
DIRECTOR, MEDICAL/SURGICAL NURSING
1. OBSTETRICS
2. PEDIATRICS
3. ORTHOPEDICS/EENT
4. MEDICAL/ONCOLOGY NURSING
5. GENERAL SURGERY, GYN, AND UROLOGY
6. GERONTOLOGY
CLINICAL SPECIALISTS
1. CARDIAC
2. PEDIATRIC
3. GERONTOLOGY
4. ENDOCRINE

FIGURE 8.1

JOB DESCRIPTION FORMAT

Position Title

Position Classification

Area:

Supervisor:

Time:

AREAS OF RESPONSIBILITY	% OF TIME	STANDARDS OF PERFORMANCE

Minimum Educational Qualifications:

Minimum Experience Qualifications:

Recommended Qualifications:

Special/Unique Position Demands:

FIGURE 11.1

TIME LOG

Department   **Position Code**   **Name**   **Date**

TIME IN 0.5 HOUR	ACTIVITIES	CATEGORY	PRIORITY LEVEL	GOAL
TIME TOTALS			H M L X	L M S

Category:

Management Process or **Nursing Process**

D = Data Collection
N = Needs/problem identification
P = Planning
Di = Directing
C = Controlling
E = Evaluation

A = Assessment
Dx = Nursing Diagnosis
P = Plan
I = Implementation
E = Evaluation

Priority Level:

H = High
M = Moderate
L = Low
X = not a priority activity

Goals:

L = Long range
M = Medium range
S = Short range

FIGURE 12.1
PODVILLE HOSPITAL PEDIATRIC UNIT

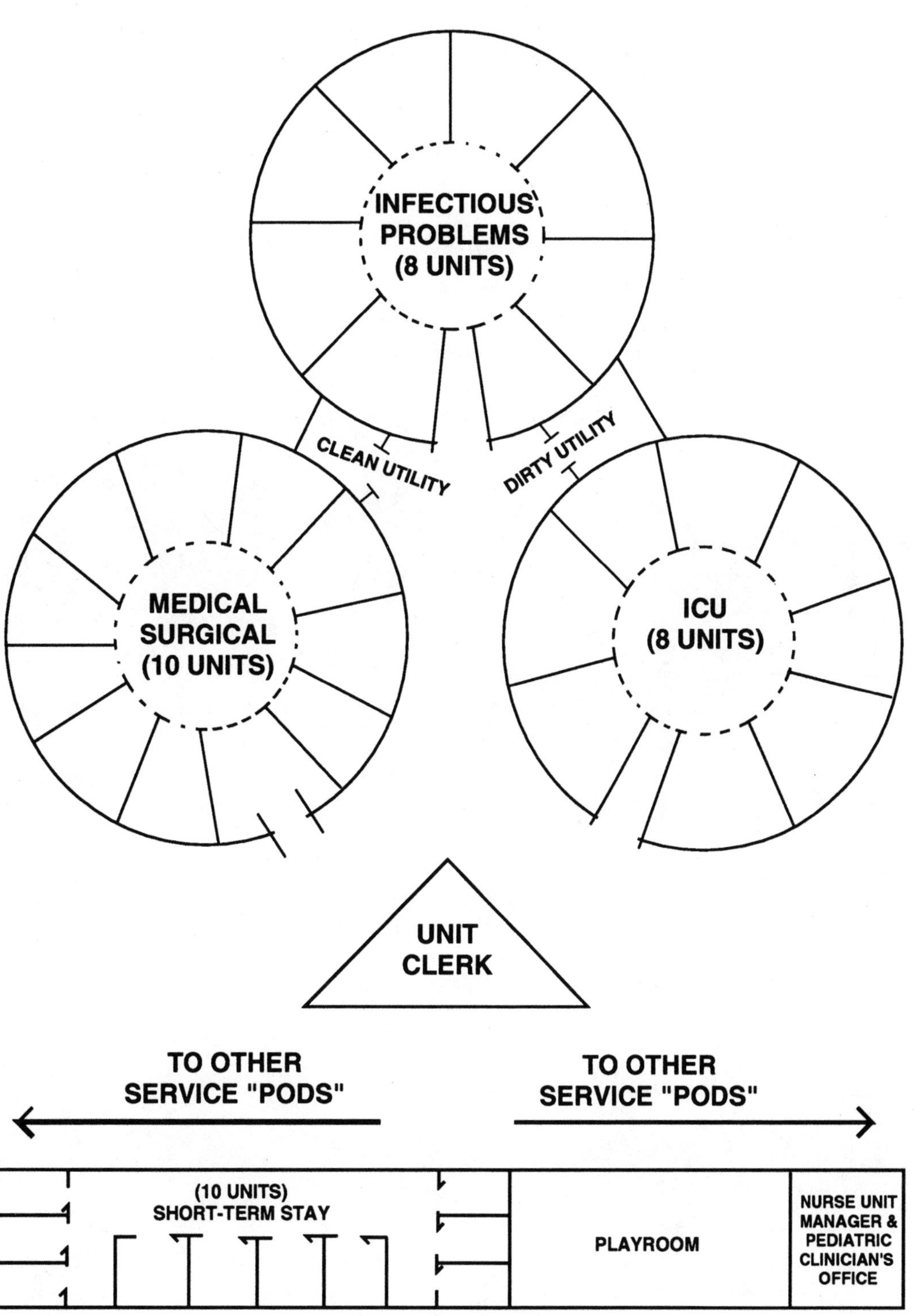

FIGURE 13.1 "OVER 70s POD"

Podville Hospital is a University Research Facility serving a retirement community which has designated product lines for the elderly for a "preferred provider" status. The modern facility is designed to accomodate diversified services.

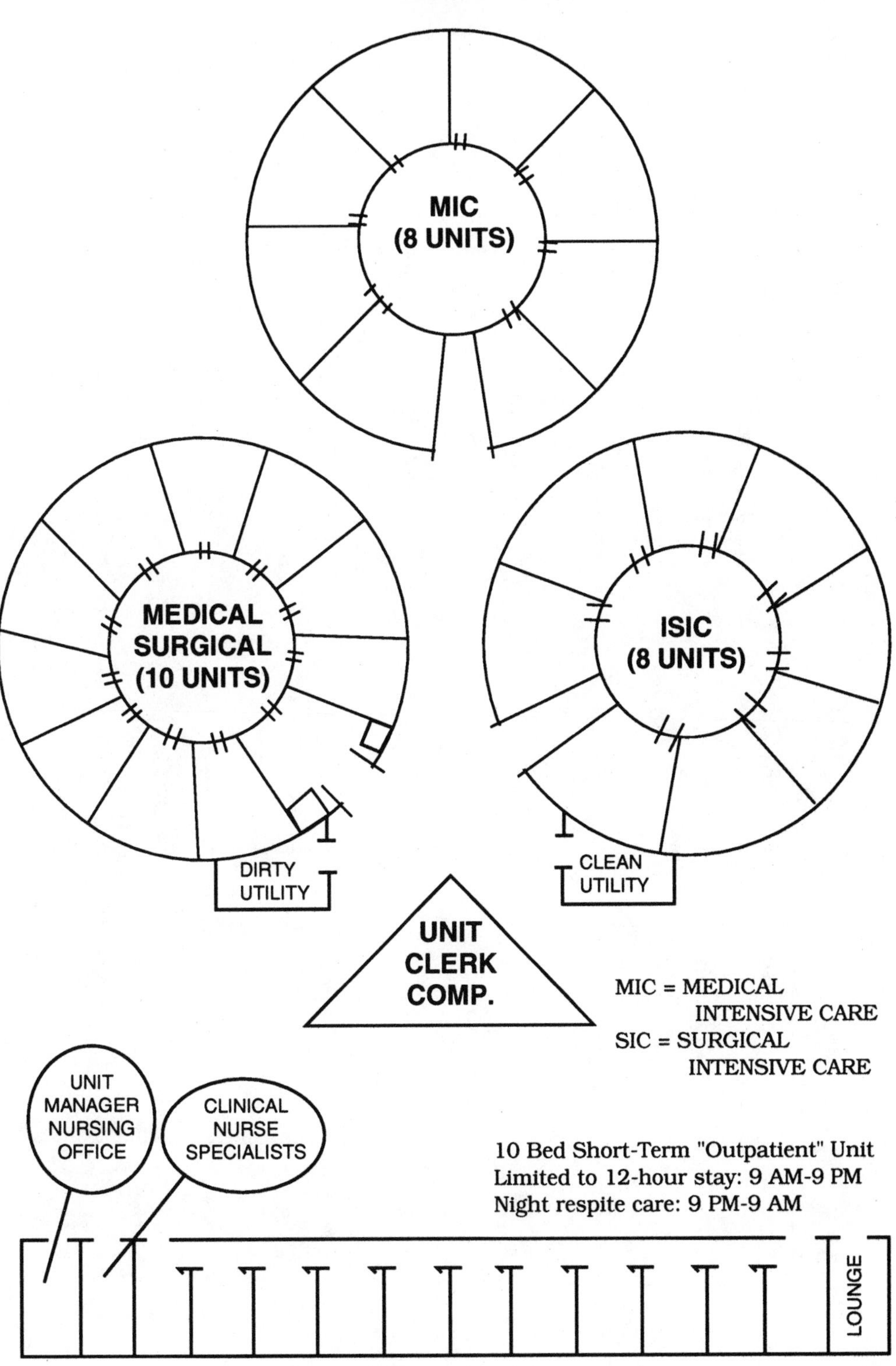

FIGURE 17.1

ANALYSIS OF STAFF TURNOVER AND STAFF REPLACEMENT

RESOURCES	STRUCTURE (Guidelines, Rules, & Policies)	PROCESS (Activities, Systems, & Procedures)	OUTCOMES (Goals, Objectives, & Standards)
Human	ex. Union contracts		
Facility		ex. Available orientation space	

FIGURE 18.1

COSTING EDUCATIONAL PROGRAMS

Program Titles: **Elective** ________ **Mandatory** ________ **Readiness Program** ________

Target Participants: ________________________ **Potential Number of Participants:** ________

If open to outsiders: Program fee ________ **Estimated reimbursement:** ________

EXPENSES

ITEM		BUDGETED	ACTUAL
0. Income			
0.1	Participant fees	______	______
0.2	Sale of program to other facilities	______	______
1. Labor Costs			
1.1	Instructor	______	______
1.2	Employee	______	______
1.3	Employee replacement	______	______
1.4	Administrative overhead	______	______
2. Educational Supplies			
2.1	Disposable supplies	______	______
2.2	Reusable supplies	______	______
2.3	Capital supplies	______	______
2.4	Media materials	______	______
3. Facility/Department Overhead			
3.1	Space/room fees	______	______
3.2	Special staff, i.e., housekeeping, security	______	______
3.3	Utilities	______	______
3.4	Depreciation	______	______
4. Marketing			
4.1	Brochures	______	______
4.2	Postage	______	______
4.3	Other	______	______
5. Refreshments			
5.1	Amount per participant x number of participants	______	______
TOTALS:		______	______
	Cost per participant	______	______

FIGURE 21.1
POWER

Self Study Sheets

Resource: Chapter 21 of text

Power is a reality. The use of power is practiced by both scrupulous and unscrupulous persons to achieve goals with which we may or may not agree. Nurse managers are wise to be aware of all types and techniques of power, whether or not all techniques of power are ones which one would chose to use within his/her own values system. Rest assured, someone will use the full repertoire of power behaviors. The following controlled notes will highlight chapter content as you study.

1. **Power is the ________________ and ________________ to influence another's behavior for the sake of producing __________ effects.**
2. **According to Buber, power is neither ___________ or _____________ within itself.**
3. **Power is ________________________ to effect change.**
4. **Controlling behavior of subordinates may be accomplished through manipulating _________________ and _____________ which are important to subordinates.**
5. **Three types of power are ________________, _______________, and ____________**
6. **Define personal power.**
7. **Define positional power.**
8. **Define social power.**

FIGURE 21.1

9. Define expert power

10. What is the difference between the need for power and the need for achievement?

11. What is the difference between direct and indirect power?

12. When is power legitimate?

13. When is power illegitimate?

14. Define:

Nutrient power:

Synergic power:

Manipulative power:

Competitive power:

Exploitive power:

FIGURE 21.1

15. Power arises out of control over ____________, ____________, and __________.

16. Why should a nurse manager seek power?

17. Power-oriented individuals:

a.

b.

18. Why do professionals in America tend to deny power?

19. Think upon this idea:

If a person does not use his/her positional power, it will be taken from him/her.

20. List six principles of power given in text. (Remember, these are statements of reality, not value statements.)

a.

b.

c.

d.

21. Give an example of each of the following basic power acquiring skills that you have seen in nursing practice.

a. Peer skills

FIGURE 21.1

b. Leadership skills

c. Informational processing skills

d. Conflict resolution skills

e. Skill in unstructured decision making

f. Entrepreneurial skills

22. The text gives many examples of the exertion and use of power. Relate four similar examples from your observations in nursing. For each example, what type of power was being used? Would you choose to copy the power behavior in the same situation? Give rationale for your answers.

FIGURE 28.1

MANAGEMENT ASSESSMENT

name ______ title ______ position ______

Area of Concern/Interest	Priority Level low 1 2 3 4 5 high	Pervasiveness 1 unit 2 multi units 3 service 4 multi services 5 hosp wide	Occurrence/ Frequency 1 yearly 2 quarterly 3 monthly 4 weekly 5 daily
Management: Structure 1. 2. 3.			
Management: Process 1. 2. 3.			
Management: Outcomes 1. 2. 3.			
Other			

FIGURE 28.2

PATIENT CARE ASSESSMENT

name ____________ title ____________ position ____________

Area of Concern/Interest	Priority Level (1 low, 2, 3, 4, 5 high)	Pervasiveness (1 unit, 2 multi units, 3 service, 4 multi services, 5 hosp wide)	Occurrence/ Frequency (1 yearly, 2 quarterly, 3 monthly, 4 weekly, 5 daily)
Patient Care: Structure 1. 2. 3.			
Patient Care: Process 1. 2. 3.			
Patient Care: Outcomes 1. 2. 3.			
Other